AF477152

Pharmaceutical Technology:
A Practical Manual

Pharmaceutical Technology:
A Practical Manual
B. Pharm and M. Pharm

Dr. Sushama Talegaonkar

Department of Pharmaceutics
Faculty of Pharmacy
Jamia Hamdard, New Delhi-62

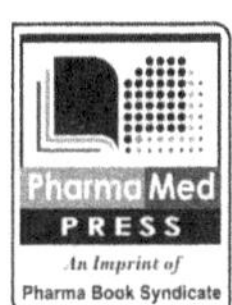

PharmaMed Press
An imprint of Pharma Book Syndicate
A unit of BSP Books Pvt. Ltd.
4-4-309/316, Giriraj Lane,
Sultan Bazar, Hyderabad - 500 095.

Pharmaceutical Technology: A Practical Manual *by*
Dr. Sushama Talegaonkar

© 2017, *by Publisher*

All rights reserved. No part of this book or parts thereof may be reproduced, stored in a retrieval system or transmitted in any language or by any means, electronic, mechanical, photocopying, recording or otherwise without the prior written permission of the publishers.

Published by

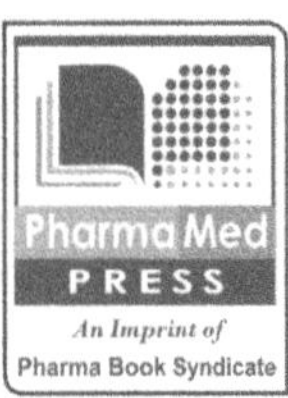

PharmaMed Press

An imprint of Pharma Book Syndicate

A unit of BSP Books Pvt. Ltd.
4-4-309/316, Giriraj Lane, Sultan Bazar, Hyderabad - 500 095.
Phone: 040-23445600, 23445688; Fax: 91+40-23445611
E-mail: info@pharmamedpress.com
www.pharmamedpress.com/pharmamedpress.net

ISBN: 978-93-5230-169-0 (Hardback)

PREFACE

Pharmaceutical technology is the science of manufacturing and evaluation of dosage forms. "Pharmaceutical Technology" is a diverse term and covers various areas like: understanding of basic physico-chemical aspects of drugs and excipients; designing of dosage form which is adequate for its purpose; manufacturing of the dosage form at small (lab) scale and large (commercial) scale; and evaluating them for the quality parameters. It also deals with the assurance of safety of the dosage form by conducting a number of quality control tests. Pharmaceutical technology has evolved from the era of manual practice to the present day complete automation and control. However, the basic principles and concepts of Pharmaceutical Technology have remained unchanged, which every pharmacy professional still needs to understand. The Pharmaceutical Technology: A Practical Manual is an attempt to establish an interface between laboratory experiments and industrial practices. This Practical Manual contains an assortment of experiments on different pharmaceutical dosage forms for better understanding of theory involved and practical implications. The book comprises of **10 chapters** and **total 31** experiments and major emphasis is given on manufacturing and evaluation of pharmaceutical dosage forms. Every chapter contains introduction, experiments followed by some questions for the self-evaluation. The book is meant for both under-graduates and post graduate pharmacy students.

The author welcomes suggestions for further improvisation in future edition.

- Author

CONTENTS

Chapter 5: Capsules 101

Experiment 18

Experiment 19

Experiment 20

Experiment 21

Chapter 6: Microencapsulation 123

Experiment 22

Chapter 7: Dispersed System 133

Experiment 23

Experiment 24

Experiment 25

Chapter 8: Aerosol 159

Chapter 9: Modified Release Drug Delivery System 183

Chapter 10: Packaging System 199

CHECKLIST FOR LABORATORY ESSENTIALS

All the students should carry the following items while entering the laboratory:

(a) Lab record notebook

(b) Rough notebook

(c) Lab apron

(d) Permanent marker

(e) Label slips

(f) Butter-paper/ weighing paper

(g) Spatula

(h) Compass box, with scale, pen and pencils.

(i) Fractional weight box

(j) Soap

(k) Scissors

(l) Glue stick

LABORATORY ETHICS

1. Always wear lab apron inside the laboratory.

2. Be familiar with your lab assignment before you come to the lab.

3. Follow good housekeeping practices. Work benches should be kept clean and tidy at all times.

4. Dispose of all chemicals, broken glass, and paper pieces into the proper containers as directed by the instructor. Do not throw them in washbasin.

5. Maintain adequate silence in laboratory and always keep your mobile phones on silent mode.

6. Never eat or drink in the laboratory.

7. Tie back all long hair and remove dangling jewellery during laboratory session.

8. Only lab notebook or lab handouts should be out on the table while performing an experiment. Books and bags should not be on the working place. Passageways need to be clear at all times.

9. Listen to the instructions of teacher or laboratory assistant carefully.

10. During weighing never place chemicals directly on the balance pan, always use butter paper or weighing bottles.

11. Always be sure that electrical equipment is turned in the "off" position before plugging it into a socket and after finishing the work.

12. Thoroughly clean your laboratory work space at the end of the laboratory session. Make sure that all equipments are clean, and returned to its original place.

13. Wash your hands properly before leaving the laboratory.

14. Report all accidents to your teacher or laboratory assistant.

MAINTENANCE OF LABORATORY NOTEBOOK

1. Make index for experiments at starting of notebook.

2. Clearly and conspicuously indicate the following information in the lab notebook:

    (i) Name of the person maintaining the notebook;

    (ii) Laboratory in which that person works;

    (iii) Starting date of the entries.

3. Be sure to record all experimental work, calculations, sketches, diagrams, and any other related information directly in the notebook.

4. It is important to make successive entries on consecutive pages. Do not insert, remove, or modify any of the pages.

5. Note down the legitimate results at the end and interpret the observations.

6. The observations in the record should be signed and dated by the teacher.

REFERENCE BOOKS
FOR WRITING THEORY OF GIVEN PRACTICALS

- Alfanso G Gennaro, Remington: The Science and Practice of Pharmacy, Lippincot Williams and Wilkins, Vol I &II, 19th Edition, 2000.
- Ansel H. C., Allen L. V. and Popovich N. G. Pharmaceutical dosage forms and drug delivery systems, Lippincott Williams Wilkins, 7th edition, 1999.
- Aulton, M. E. Pharmaceutics: The science of dosage form design, ELBS Publisher, Churchill Livingstone, UK, 1st Edition 1988.
- Banker, G.S. and Rhodes, C.T. Modern Pharmaceutics, Marcel Dekker, Inc., New York, Vol 40, 2nd Edition, 1990.
- Beringer, P., et al. Remington: The science and practice of Pharmacy, Vol 1 and 2, 21st Edition, Philadelphia College of Pharmacy and Science. Philadelphia, PA, 2006.
- Brahmankar, D. M. and Jaiswal, S. B. Biopharmaceutics and Pharmacokinetics – A Treatise, Vallabh Prakashan, 1st edition, 1999.
- Brody, A. L. and Marsh, K. S. Encyclopedia of Packaging Technology, 2nd Edition, John Wiley and Sons Inc., 1997.
- Chien, Y. Novel Drug Delivery Systems, Marcel Dekker, Inc., New York, Vol 14, 2nd Edition, 1987.
- Cooper and Gunn's Tutorial Pharmacy, CBS Publishers and Distributors, 6th Edition, 1999.
- Gibson, M. Pharmaceutical preformulation and formulation: A practical guide from candidate drug selection to commercial dosage form, Vol 199, Informa Healthcare, New York, USA, 2009.
- Indian Pharmacopoeia. Vol 1-3, New Delhi: Ministry of Health and Family Welfare, Government of India, Controller of Publication. 2012.
- Jain, N. K. Advances in controlled and novel drug delivery system, CBS Publishers and Distributors, 1st Edition, 2001.
- Krowezynski, L. Extended Release Dosage Forms, CRC Press, Inc., Boca Raton, 1987.

- Kydonieus, A. Treatise on controlled drug delivery: Fundamentals/ optimization/applications, Marcel Dekker, Inc., New York, 1991.
- Lachman, L., Liberman, H. A. and Kanig, J. L. Theory and practices of Industrial Pharmacy, Varghese publishing house, 3rd Edition, 1987.
- Liberman, H. A., Lachman, L. and Schwartz, J. B. Pharmaceutical dosage forms: Tablets, Marcel Dekker Inc, New York, Vol. 1, 2 and 3, 2nd Edition 1989.
- Mathiowitz, E. Encyclopedia of Controlled Drug Delivery, John Wiley and Sons Inc., Vol I and Vol II, 1999.
- Robinson, J. R. and Lee, V.L.H. Controlled drug delivery: Fundamentals and applications, Marcel Dekker, Inc., New York, Vol 29, 2nd Edition, 1987.
- Subrahmanyam, CVS, Pharmaceutical engineering, Vallabh Prakashan Publishers. 199-257.
- Swarbrick, J. and Boylan, J. C. Encyclopedia of Pharmaceutical Technology, Marcel Dekker Inc, New York, Vol 2, 3, 4, 6, 7, 9, 12, 14, 1988.
- Talegaonkar, S., Khar, R.K., Ahmad, F. J. and Iqbal, Z.I. Pharmaceutical Technology, Birla Publication, Vol I, 1st edition, 2006-07.
- United States Pharmacopoeia. The official Compendia of standard USP 27/NF 22, Asian edition, United States Pharmaceutical Convention Inc, 2004.

HOW TO WRITE AN EXPERIMENT?

I. Things to be written on the left hand side (left page) of the practical record:

    (a) Formula

    (b) Sketches/figures (if any)

    (c) Observations

    (d) Calculation

II. Things to be written on the right hand side (right page) of the practical record:

    (a) Object

    (b) References

    (c) Requirements

    (d) Principle/ Theory

    (e) Procedure

    (f) Precautions

    (g) Results

1
Mixing

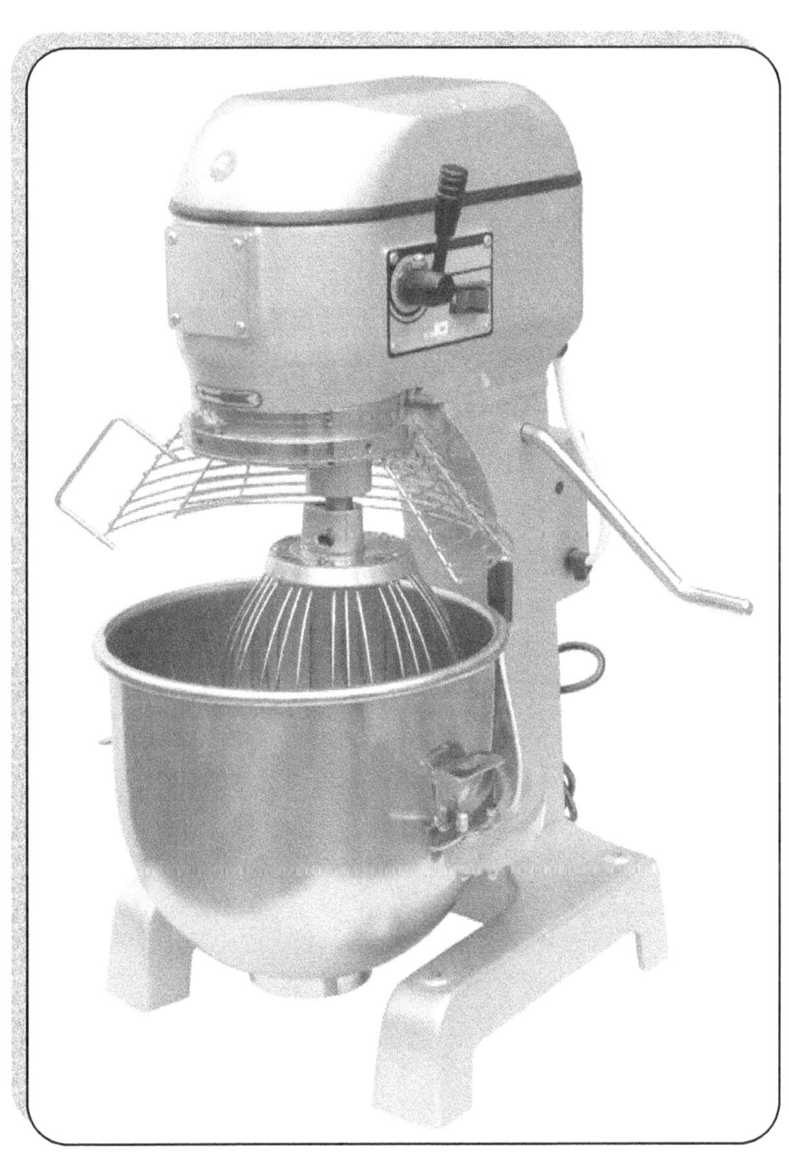

Mixing may be defined as a unit operation that aims to treat two or more components, initially in an unmixed or partially mixed state, so that each unit (particle, molecule etc.) of the components lies as nearly as possible in contact with a unit of each of the other components.

TYPES OF MIXTURES

Mixtures may be categorized into three types.

Positive mixtures: Positive mixtures are formed from materials such as gases or miscible liquids which mix *spontaneously* **and** *irreversibly* by diffusion, and tend to approach a perfect mix. There is no input of energy required with positive mixtures if the time available for mixing is unlimited, although it will shorten the time required to obtain the desired degree of mixing. In general, materials that mix by positive mixing present no problems during product manufacture.

Negative mixtures: With negative mixtures the components will tend to separate out. If this occurs quickly, then energy must be continuously provided to keep the components adequately dispersed, e.g., with a suspension formulation, such as calamine lotion, where there is a dispersion of solids in a liquid of low viscosity. With other negative mixtures the components tend to separate very slowly, e.g., emulsions, creams and viscous suspensions. Negative mixtures are generally more difficult to form and maintain and require a higher degree of mixing efficiency than do positive mixtures.

Neutral mixtures: Neutral mixtures are said to be static in behavior, i.e., the components have no tendency to mix spontaneously or segregate spontaneously once work has been input to mix them. Examples of this type of mixture include mixed powders, pastes and ointments. It should be noted that the type of mixture might change during processing. For example, if the viscosity increases the mixture may change from a negative to a neutral mixture. Similarly, if the particle size, degree of wetting or liquid surface tension changes the mixture type may also change.

Factors affecting solid-solid mixing
(a) Material density
(b) Particle size and distribution
(c) Wettability
(d) Stickiness/Moisture content

    (e)   Particle shape/roughness
    (f)   Selection of mixer

APPLICATIONS

To ensure the uniformity of dose.

Mechanisms of Mixing

Mixing involves the following steps:

- Convective movement of relatively large portions of the bed (Macromixing)
- Shear failure, which reduces the scale of segregation
- Diffusive movement of individual particles (Micromixing).

Evaluation of powder mixture: Mixing process is critically affected by a multitude of parameters like mixing time, mechanism of mixing, type of mixer and batch size. Various methods have been developed to quantify the quality of mixture.

Mixing Index

There is always some variation in the composition of the samples drawn from a random mixture and the standard deviation in the composition of large number of such samples can be determined, provided an accurate assay method is available. A random mix gives samples with low standard deviation as compared to mixture of the same components that have not reached the random state. This phenomenon is used to define mixing index, which is expressed as,

$$M = \frac{S_r}{S_{act}}$$

where, S_r is the Standard deviation of samples drawn from a fully random mix

S_{act} is actual Standard deviation determined on the partially mixed system.

SCALE OF SCRUTINY

Danckwert established the concept of scale of scrutiny which describes the minimum size of the regions of segregation in a particular mixture which would cause it to be regarded as insufficiently mixed. A poor mixture will have large scale of segregation and high intensity of segregation and vice versa. As the scale and intensity of the mixture is reduced the mixture passes from a stage of being unsatisfactory to satisfactory mixture.

Equipments: The detailed classification of the equipments used in soli-solid mixing is given below.

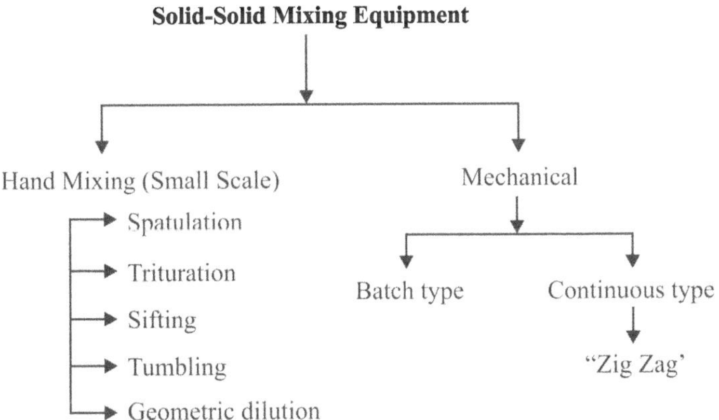

BATCH TYPE (LARGE SCALE)

(A) Batch types

I. Rotation of entire mixer shell or body with no agitator or mixing blade.

    (a) Barrel

    (b) Cube

    (c) V. shaped

    (d) Double cone

    (e) Slant double cone

II. Rotation of the entire mixer shell or body with a rotating high shear agitator blade.

    (a) V. shaped

    (b) Double cone

III. Stationary shell or body with a rotating mixing blade.

    (a) Ribbon

    (b) Sigma blade

    (c) Planetary

    (d) Conical screw

IV. High speed granulations (stationary shell or body with a rotating mixing blade and high speed agitator blade)

    (a) Barrel

    (b) Bowl

V. Air mixer (stationary shell or body, moving air as agitator)

    (a) Fluid bed granulator

    (b) Fluid bed dryer

(B) Continuous types

    I. Barrel

    II. Zigzag

1

To Perform Mixing of Solid in a Solid by Double Cone Blender and Evaluate the Quality of Mixing

Requirements: Double cone blender, drug, diluents, test tubes, Plastic beakers, Pipette, Volumetric flasks, spatula, UV spectrophotometer, UV quartz cells, funnel.

Reference: Refer any book given in the list of books at the beginning of this manual.

Principle

Double cone blenders are versatile machines used for mixing dry powder and granules homogeneously. These machines have a cylindrical shell with two conical frustums provided with opening for charging and discharging. The mixing vessel rotates along its horizontal axis. The mixing in double cone blender works by diffusion. Speed and time of rotation significantly affects the quality of mixing. All the contact

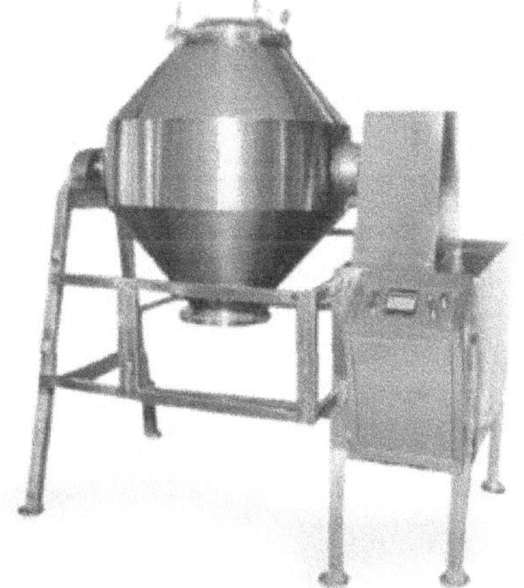

Fig. 1.1 Double cone mixer.

parts are made from superior grade of stainless steel. Double cone blenders find extensive application in Pharmaceutical, Food, Chemical and Cosmetic industries.

Procedure

- Make a standard plot of the drug (as mentioned in dissolution experiments) in a suitable solvent in which drug and diluents should be soluble.
- Take 50 mg of the given drug in a 250 mL plastic beaker.
- Add 5 g of the chosen diluent in the beaker.
- Withdraw small quantity of the mixture from different corners (top, medium, bottom) of the bulk kept in the beaker at 0 minute.
- Fix the beaker in a double cone blender and switch on the blender.
- Withdraw small quantity of the mixture from different corners (top, medium, bottom) of the bulk kept in the beaker at different time intervals 2, 4, 6, 8 and 10 minutes.
- Weight the 10 mg material from each withdrawn sample and dissolve in a suitable vehicle (in which the drug and diluent is soluble and standard plot of drug was prepared) in a volumetric flask and make the dilutions as per the requirement.
- Take the absorbance of the samples and calculate the quantity of the drug from the linear equation obtained from the standard plot.
- The time at which all three samples show same concentration taken as a ideal mixing time

Observations and Calculations

Table 1.1 Standard plot of the drug

S. No.	Concentration (µg/mL)	Absorbance
1	2	
2	4	
3	6	
4	8	
5	10	
6	12	
7	14	

Formula

$$\% \text{ Drug} = \frac{\text{Conc. of drug (µg/mL)} \times \text{dilution factor} \times \text{total volume}}{\text{total weight}} \times 100$$

Table 1.2 Analysis of samples collected at different time intervals

S. No.	Time (mins)	Concentration of drug present (µg/mL)			Inference
		Sample 1	Sample 2	Sample 3	
1	0				**Poor/Good/Excellent Mixing**
2	2				
3	4				
4	6				
5	8				
6	10				

Results: The effective time for proper mixing of the given drug with the diluent was found to be _________ minutes.

Precautions

1. Before mixing, mixer should be cleaned and check for any drug residue of previous batches.
2. Ideal mixer should be selected for the purpose.

PHARMA TRIVIA: SELF EVALUATION TEST

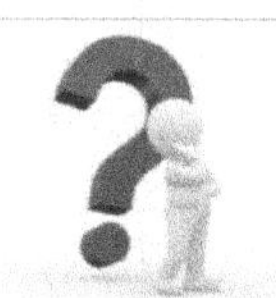

1. Define mixing.
2. What do you mean by degree of mixing?
3. What are the different types of mixtures?
4. Enlist the factors affecting solid-solid mixing.
5. Enlist the factors affecting liquid-liquid mixing.
6. Enlist the factors affecting mixing of semi-solids.
7. Enumerate the mechanisms of mixing of fluids.
8. Write down the mechanisms of solid- solid mixing.
9. Give examples of any two equipments used in semisolid mixing.
10. Give examples of equipments used for solid mixing.
11. Give examples of any two equipments used for liquid mixing.
12. Give the working principle of double cone mixer.
13. What do you mean by vortexing?
14. What do you understand by turbulent mixing?
15. Explain in brief shear mixing?
16. Briefly explain convective mixing.
17. What do you understand by molecular diffusion?
18. Define the terms: positive, negative and neutral mixing.
19. Define the term intensity of segregation and scale of segregation.
20. Differentiate between the terms macro mixing and micro mixing.

2
Dissolution

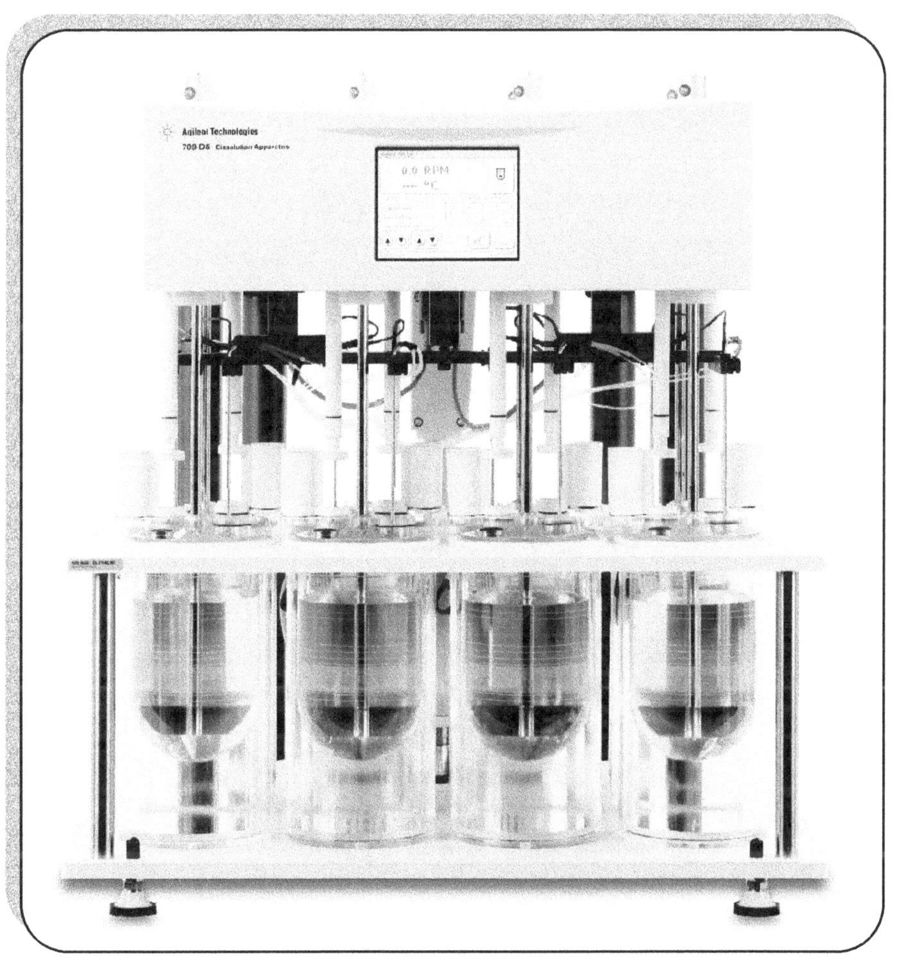

Dissolution is the process by which a solute forms a **solution in a solvent.** The solute, in the case of solids, has its crystalline structure disintegrated as separate ions, atoms, and molecules form. For liquids and gases, the molecules must be adaptable with those of the solvent for a solution to form. Dissolution testing is widely used in the pharmaceutical industry for optimization of formulation and quality control.

The rate at which solute dissolves in solvent (Dissolution rate) depends on:

- Nature of the solvent and solute
- Temperature (and to a small extent pressure)
- Degree of undersaturation
- Presence of mixing device
- Interfacial surface area
- Presence of inhibitors (e.g., a substance adsorbed on the surface).

Many devices have been reported for determination of the dissolution rate. The procedures differ in degree rather than in basic principle. The conditions common to the most *in-vitro* dissolution tests are

- The use of simulated gastric and intestinal fluid at $37 \pm 2\ ^{\circ}C$.
- The use of a device for agitating the element and product at a fixed speed.
- The use of a screen for separating disintegrated particles from the bulk of the product.
- The time intervals, composition of the fluids, type of agitator and mesh size of the screen are the usual variant in the methods.

CLASSIFICATION OF DISSOLUTION TESTING DEVICES

Dissolution-rate methods may be classified according to a variety of factors. Where the surface area of a pure drug is held constant, the intrinsic dissolution rate of the drug is measured in terms of amount of drug released per unit area and per unit time. The agitation intensity offers another alternative for classification, since alteration of the stationary film thickness surrounding the dissolution particles is reflected in a change in the dissolution-rate constant. Thus the methods may be classified depending on the nature of flow of the dissolution medium with respect to the dissolving substrate. Accordingly, the classification can be as follows.

- Methods exhibiting natural-convection flow characteristics
- Methods exhibiting forced-convection streamline-flow characteristics
- Methods exhibiting forced-convection turbulent-flow characteristics

Table 2.1 summarizes various types and uses of different dissolution apparatus.

Table 2.1 Application of various dissolution Apparatus

Type of Apparatus	Name of Apparatus	Dosage form Evaluated
Type I	Basket apparatus	Solid dosage form (Immediate release, Modified release Products), chewable Tablets
Type II	Paddle apparatus	
Type III	Reciprocating cylinder	Extended release drug products
Type IV	Flow through cell apparatus	Drug products that contain active ingredients with limited solubility
Type V	Paddle over disk	Suppositories, poorly soluble drugs, implants, transdermal patch.
Type VI	Rotating Cylinder	Transdermal dosage form
Type VII	Reciprocating holder	Non disintegrating oral modified dosage form as well as traditional dosage form

As per IP: Two types of apparatus are specified

1. Apparatus 1 (Paddle apparatus)
2. Apparatus 2 (Basket apparatus)

As per USP: Seven types of apparatus are specified

1. Apparatus 1 (Basket apparatus)
2. Apparatus 2 (Paddle apparatus)
3. Apparatus 3 (Reciprocating cylinder)
4. Apparatus 4 (Flow through cell)
5. Apparatus 5 (Paddle over disk)
6. Apparatus 6 (Rotating cylinder)
7. Apparatus 7 (Reciprocating holder)

2

To Study the Various Types of Dissolution Apparatus

Requirements: Various types of Dissolution apparatus.

Reference: Refer any book given in the list of book at the beginning of this manual.

TYPES OF APPARATUS

I Apparatus 1 (Basket Apparatus)

- Basket apparatus was the first official method. Essentially it consisted of an approximately 1 inch (25.4 mm) × 13/8 inch (34.925 mm) stainless steel, 40-mesh wire basket rotated at a constant speed between 25 and 150 rpm (Fig. 2.1). This method is now called Apparatus 1.

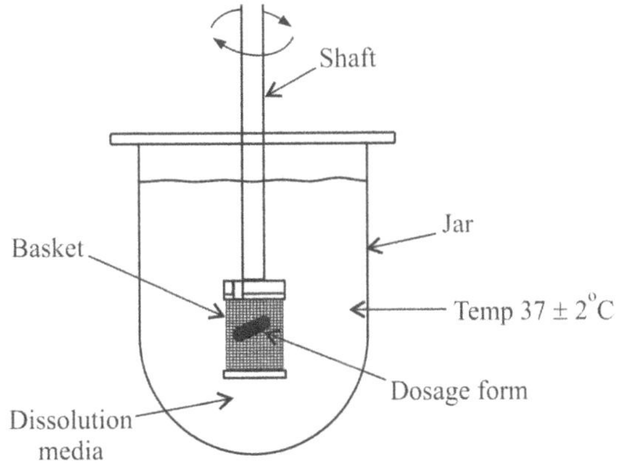

Fig. 2.1 Basket apparatus.

- The apparatus consists of a metallic drive shaft connected to the cylindrical basket. The basket is positioned inside a vessel made of glass or other inert, transparent material. The temperature inside the vessel is kept at a constant value by being placed inside a water bath or heating jacket. The solution in the vessel is stirred smoothly by the rotating stirring element.

- A speed-regulating device is used that allows the shaft rotation speed to be selected and maintained at a specified rate, within ± 4 %.

- Shaft and basket components of the stirring element are fabricated of stainless steel.

- The distance between the inside bottom of the vessel and the bottom of the basket is maintained at 25 ± 2 mm during the test.

- Other types of baskets exist for specific applications, for example, suppository baskets are normally manufactured from plastic and have vertical slits to facilitate the dissolution.

- This apparatus is used mainly for testing of uncoated tablets, enteric coated tablets, sublingual tablets, hard gelatin capsules and soft gelatin capsules.

II Apparatus 2 (Paddle Type) (Fig. 2.2)

- The USP specifies that the paddle must rotate smoothly without significant wobble. The arc of the paddle blade creates considerable flow and wobbles and has the effect of increasing the angular velocity at the paddle tips in a manner that couples with the fluid much more signifycantly than would a comparable wobble in the basket.

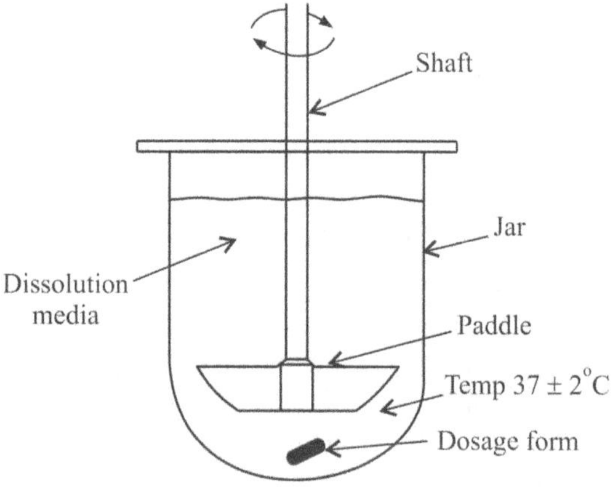

Fig. 2.2 Paddle apparatus.

- The contours of the paddle blade must not include any sharp edges at the tips for that could produce turbulent instead of laminar flow patterns. The USP constrains wobble and vertical alignment with the axis of the vessel to be, within ± 2.0 mm.

- The USP suggests that paddles 'may be' coated with polyfluorocarbon and most commercial paddles are accordingly coated. Such coating serves two purposes: it prevents corrosion and the introduction of unwanted ions into the media and it seals the joint where the blade is attached to the shaft, thus preventing the accumulation of traces of contaminants.

- The stirring paddle has been specified as a stainless steel device rather than a glass one with a detachable blade, because of the precise geometry required for the repeatability of the paddle method, and also the glass cannot be manufactured to such close cost specifications without incurring excessive cost.

- Rotation speed for solid dosage forms is 50 rpm, while for liquid dosage forms (suspension) it is 25 rpm.

- It cannot be used for testing of powder dosage forms.

- This apparatus is used mainly for testing of uncoated tablets, enteric coated tablets, sublingual tablets, hard gelatin capsules and soft gelatin capsules, gels, ointments.

III Apparatus 3 (Reciprocating Cylinder)

The assembly consists of:

- A set of cylindrical, flat-bottomed glass vessels;

- A set of glass reciprocating cylinders.

- Inert fittings (stainless steel type 316 or other suitable material).

- Screens that are made of suitable nonsorbing and nonreactive material, and that are designed to fit the tops and bottoms of the reciprocating cylinders.

- A motor and drive assembly to reciprocate the cylinders vertically inside the vessels.

- The vessels are partially immersed in a suitable water-bath of any convenient size that permits holding the temperature at 37 ± 0.5 °C during the test.

- A device is used that allows the reciprocation rate to be selected and maintained at the specified dip rate, within ± 5 %.

- This apparatus resembles the disintegration apparatus.

- Upward and downward strokes of cylinder are observed.

- It is quite useful for beaded products like pellets, granules etc., and also useful for controlled and immediate release products.

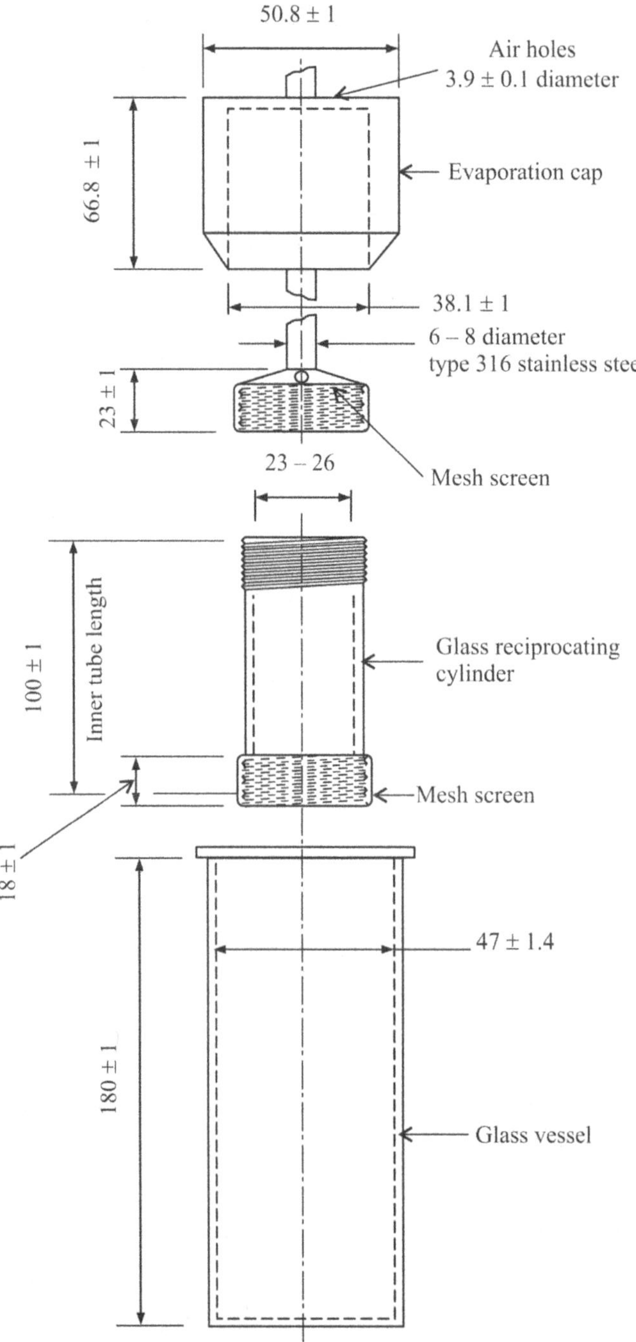

Fig. 2.3 Reciprocating cylinder (U.S.P.).

IV Apparatus 4 (Flow through Cell)

The assembly consists of

- A pump for the dissolution medium;

- A flow-through cell;

- A water-bath to maintain the dissolution medium at $37 \pm 0.5°C$.

- The pump forces the dissolution medium upwards through the flow-through cell. The pump has a delivery range between 240 mL/h and 960 mL/h, with standard flow rates of 4 mL/min, 8 mL/min, and 16 mL/min. It must deliver a constant flow ($\pm$ 5 % of the nominal flow rate).

- The flow-through cell of transparent and inert material is mounted verti-

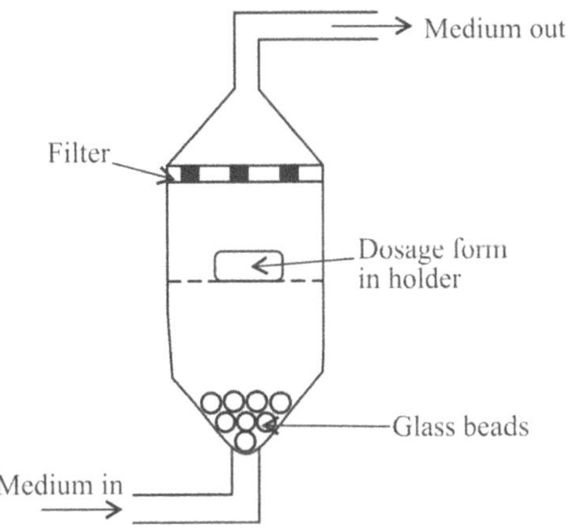

Fig. 2.4 Flow through cell.

cally, with a filter system that prevents escape of undissolved particles from the top of the cell; standard cell diameters are 12 mm and 22.6 mm; the bottom cone is usually filled with small glass beads of about 1 mm diameter, with 1 bead of about 5 mm positioned at the apex to protect the fluid entry tube; a tablet holder is available for positioning of special dosage forms. The cell is immersed in a water-bath, and the temperature is maintained at 37 ± 0.5 °C

- It is mainly used for testing of sugar coated tablets, suppositories, semisolid dosage forms, powder, granules, and implants.

V Apparatus 5 (Paddle Over Disk)

- Transdermal patch testing is carried out using USP method 5 (paddle over disc).

- With paddle over disc, the transdermal patch is placed between a glass disc and an inert PTFE (Poly Teflon) mesh.

- This is placed at the bottom of the vessel, with the mesh facing upwards, under a rotating paddle.

- Unlike dissolution testing, transdermal testing is carried out at 32 °C to reflect the lower temperature of the skin. Other variables such as the height setting and sampling requirements are the same as dissolution testing.

- USP apparatus 5 is made-up of borosilicate glass with a PTFE 17 mesh, held together by PTFE clips. Patches up to 90 mm in diameter can be tested.

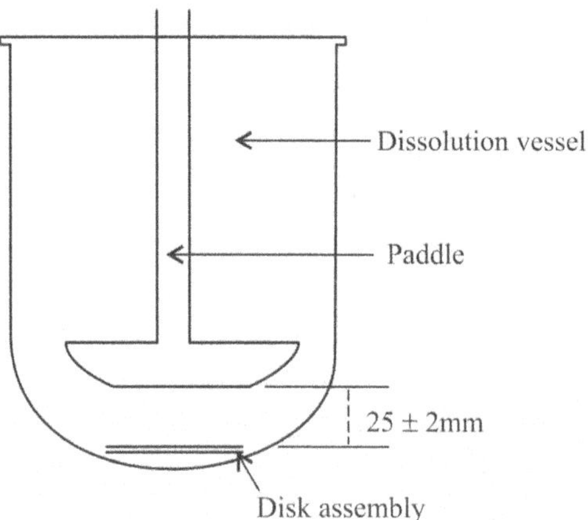

Fig. 2.5 Paddle over disk.

VI Apparatus 6 (Rotating Cylinder)

- Transdermal or patch testing is carried out using USP method 5 (paddle over disc) or USP method 6, the rotating cylinder.

- The rotating cylinder is very similar to USP method 1 (the rotating basket).

- With USP method 6 however, the basket assembly is replaced by a solid stainless steel cylinder.

- The cylinder consists of two parts that fit together:

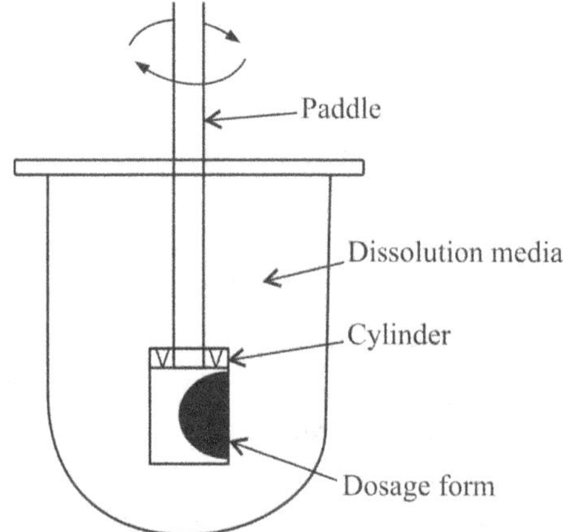

Fig. 2.6 Rotating cylinder.

the main shaft/cylinder assembly plus an extension. The extension is used when the transdermal patch requires a larger area.

- The distance between the inside bottom of the vessel and the cylinder is maintained at 25 ± 2 mm during the test.

- The temperature is maintained at 32 ± 0.5 °C. The vessel is covered during the test to minimize evaporation.

VII Apparatus 7 (Reciprocating Holder)

- The vessels are partially immersed in a suitable water-bath of any convenient size that permits holding the temperature at 37 ± 0.5 °C during the test.

- A device is used that allows the reciprocation rate to be selected and maintained at the specified dip rate, within ± 5 % limit.

- Useful for testing of extended release dosage forms, osmotic pumps, tablets, ointments, gels etc.

- Cuprophan (Cellophane paper) is used for holding of semisolid dosage forms.

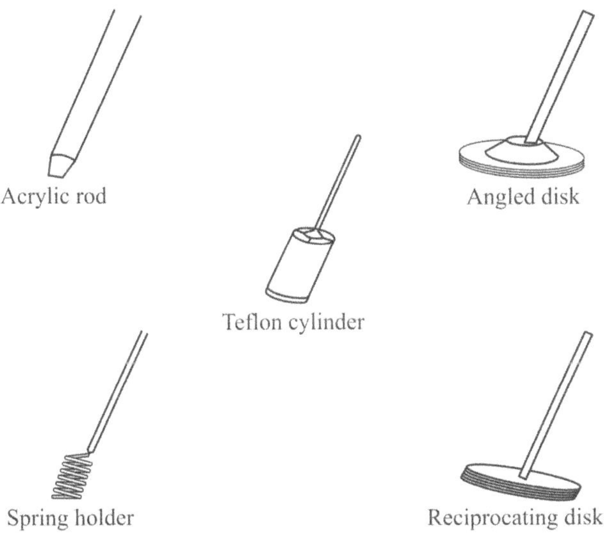

Fig. 2.7 Reciprocating holder.

Results: The diagrams, working principles and applications were studied for different dissolution apparatus.

3

To Study the *In Vitro* Dissolution Profile of Conventional Paracetamol Tablet

Requirements: Volumetric flask, beakers, test tubes, UV spectro-photometer, UV quartz cells, volumetric flasks, dissolution apparatus (Paddle type), pipette, funnel, filter paper, drug sample etc.

Reference: Refer any book given in the list of books at the beginning of this manual.

Principle

Dissolution is defined as a physicochemical process by which a solid chemical or a drug substance dissolves in the solvent phase to yield a solution. In biologic system dissolution is an important prerequisite for any orally administered drug to be systemically effective. In an oral dosage form, release properties are mainly affected by disintegration of solid substance into granules, deaggregation of granules to form fine particles and dissolution of drug from fine particles into solution. Rate of drug dissolution is given by **Noyes Whitney equation**:

$$dc/dt = DA(C_s\text{-}C)h$$

where, dc/dt – Rate of drug dissolution

D- Diffusion rate constant

A-Surface area of particles

C_s- Drug conc. in stagnant layer

C- Drug conc. in bulk solvent

h- Thickness of hydrodynamic boundary layer

Immediate or conventional release dosage forms (IR) are those which deliver drug rapidly into blood circulation. Dissolution studies for IR dosage form are done using USP apparatus 1-4. Dissolution test is performed by adding stated volume of dissolution medium into vessel of apparatus and warming it to 36.5-37.5 °C.

Note: Typical USP requirement for IR dosage form are that 75% of active ingredient from dosage form should be dissolve in water or acid at 37 °C in 45 minutes in USP 1 or 2 apparatus.

Procedure

Step I: Preparation of calibration curve

1. Accurately weigh 10 mg of drug reference and transfer it into a 100 mL volumetric flask through funnel.
2. Dissolve the drug in distilled water and make up the volume up to 100 mL (stock solution).
3. Take 0.2, 0.4, 0.6, 0.8, 1, 1.2, 1.4, 1.6, 1.8 and 2 mL of stock to the 10 mL volumetric flask separately and make up the volume up to 10 mL with distilled water.
4. Clean the quartz cells by rinsing them with distilled water.
5. Add blank solution (dilution media) to both the cells and do base line correction.
6. Replace the blank solution from one of the cells with drug dilution and carry out the spectrum analysis from 200- 800 nm.
7. Obtain the λ_{max} for the drug and use the wavelength for further absorption readings.
8. Again add blank solution (dilution media) to both the cell and set auto zero at λ_{max} obtained in step 7.
9. Replace the solution from one of the cells with drug dilutions prepared in step 3, and record the absorption readings.
10. Draw a graph between absorbance (Y axis) and concentration (X axis) to obtain the calibration curve.

Note: Use methanol or Sodium lauryl sulphate solution as per requirement for solubilization of drug.

Step II: Dissolution study

1. Clean the vessel and place 900 mL of deareated dissolution medium (distilled water or 0.1 N HCl) in the vessel of apparatus I (I.P.) and set temperature at 37 ± 2 °C.

2. Place one tablet in the vessel and operate the rotation of paddle at 50 rpm.

3. Withdraw the 5 mL sample from zone midway between the surface of dissolution medium and the top of the rotating paddle at the defined time intervals (5, 10, 15, 20 30, and 45 min).

4. Add 5 mL of fresh dissolution media at time of each withdrawal.

5. Filter the sample, make the proper dilutions (if needed) and measure the absorbance of samples by using UV spectrophotometer at respective λ_{max}.

6. Calculate concentration of drug using calibration curve.

7. Calculate the cumulative amount of drug released at different points using the following equation.

Cumulative amount drug released = Concentration (μg/mL) $\times$ 900 $\times$ Dilution factor / Labeled amount of drug

8. Construct the drug release profile by taking the cumulative amount of drug released on the y-axis and time on the x-axis.

Observations

Table 3.1 Data of dissolution test of Paracetamol

Time (min)	Absorbance (nm)	Concentration of diluted solution (mg/mL)	Dilution factor	Amount released (mg)
0				
5				
10				
15				
20				
30				
45				
60				

Calculations

Cumulative amount drug released = Concentration (μg/mL) $\times$ 900 $\times$ Dilution factor / Labeled amount of drug

Results: ________mg of drug was released in ________minutes. Maximum amount of drug (C_{max}) was found to be ________at ________minute (T_{max}).

Precautions

1. Apparatus should be properly cleaned.
2. Sample should be filtered through Whatman filter paper before UV analysis.

4

To Study the Dissolution Profile of Modified Release Tablet (Enteric Coated Tablet)

Requirements: Volumetric flask, beakers, test tubes, UV spectrophotometer, UV quartz cells, dissolution apparatus (Basket), pipette, funnel, filter paper, drug sample, dissolution medium (**Phosphate buffer pH 6.8 or 7.4 I.P.**).

Reference: Refer any book given in the list of books at the beginning of this manual.

Principle

Intrinsic dissolution of a pure substance is the rate at which it dissolves from constant surface area keeping temperature, pH, agitation and ionic strength of dissolution medium constant. Dissolution Mechanism involves heterogeneous reactions which includes overall mass transfer process to take place in 2 steps:

(a) Diffusion limited model i.e., convective transport of soluble drug through hydrodynamic boundary layers surrounding solid-liquid interphase to bulk phase.

(b) Reaction limited model i.e., interfacial transport at solid-liquid interphase.

Modified release dosage form are those which by virtue of formulation and product design, provide drug release in a modified form, distinct from that of conventional dosage form. It includes Delayed or

Extended release dosage form. Delayed action tablet dosage form is intended to release drug after sometime delay or after tablet has passed through one part of the G.I.T. to another. eg., Enteric coated tablet which are designed to pass through stomach unaltered to release the drug within intestine. Some of the polymers used to obtain enteric coating are Cellulose acetate phthalate, HPMC phthalate, PVA phthalate. While Extended release dosage forms release drug slowly, so that plasma concentrations are maintained at a therapeutic level for a prolonged period of time (usually between 8 and 12 hours).

The rate of drug release from an MR dosage form varies according to the particular formulation technique employed. Consequently, depending on the degree of control over release, MR products are generally designed to provide either:

1. The prompt achievement of a plasma concentration of drug that remains constant at a value within the therapeutic range of the drug for a prolonged period of time, or

2. The prompt achievement of a plasma concentration of drug which, although not remaining constant, declines at such a slow rate that the plasma concentration remains within the therapeutic range for a prolonged period of time.

Procedure

Step I: Preparation of calibration curve

1. Accurately weigh 10 mg of drug reference and transfer it into a 100 mL volumetric flask through funnel.

2. Dissolve the drug in Phosphate buffer pH 7.4 (IP) or pH 6.8 (IP) and make up the volume up to 100 ml (stock solution).

3. Take 0.2, 0.4, 0.6, 0.8, 1, 1.2, 1.4, 1.6, 1.8 and 2 mL of stock to the 10 mL volumetric flask separately and make up the volume up to 10 mL with Phosphate buffer.

4. Clean the quartz cells by rinsing them with Phosphate buffer.

5. Add blank solution (dilution media) to both the cells and do base line correction.

6. Replace the blank solution from one of the cells with drug dilution and carry out the spectrum analysis from 200- 800 nm.

7. Obtain the λ_{max} for the drug and use the wavelength for further absorption readings.

8. Again add blank solution (dilution media) to both the cell and set auto zero at λ_{max} obtained in step 7.

9. Replace the solution from one of the cells with drug dilutions prepared in step 3, and record the absorption readings after 24 hrs.

10. Draw a graph between absorption (Y axis) and concentration (X axis) to obtain the calibration curve.

Note: Use methanol or Sodium lauryl sulphate solution as per requirement for solubilization of drug.

Step II. Dissolution study

1. Clean the vessel and place 900 mL of deareated dissolution medium (Phosphate buffer pH 7.4 (IP) or pH 6.8 (IP) in the vessel of apparatus I (I.P.) and set temperature at $37 \pm 2\ ^\circ C$.

2. Place one tablet in the vessel and operate the rotation of paddle at 50 rpm.

3. Withdraw the 5 mL sample from zone midway between the surface of dissolution medium and the top of the rotating paddle at the defined time intervals (5, 10, 15, 20 30 and 45 min).

4. Add 5 mL of fresh dissolution media at time of each withdrawal.

5. Filter the sample, make the proper dilutions (if needed) and measure the absorbance of samples by using UV spectrophotometer at respective λ_{max}.

6. Calculate concentration of drug using calibration curve.

7. Calculate the cumulative amount of drug released at different points using the following equation.

Cumulative amount drug released = Concentration ($\mu g/mL$) $\times$ 900 $\times$ Dilution factor / Labeled amount of drug

8. Construct the drug release profile by taking the cumulative amount of drug released on the y-axis and time on the x-axis.

Note: As per USP for Modified release dosage form, a dissolution profile data would be generated at a no. of time points (5) until either 80% of the drug is release or dissolution profile reach an asymptote.

Observations and Calculations

Same as previous experiment.

Table 4.1 Dissolution data of diclofenac tablet in phosphate buffer pH 7.4

Time (Hrs)	Absorbance (nm)	Concentration of diluted solution (mg/mL)	Dilution factor	Amount released (mg)
0				
0.5				
1				
2				
3				
4				
5				
6				
7				
8				
12				
18				
24				

Results: _______ mg of drug was released in _______ minutes.

Precautions

Same as previous experiment.

5

To Compare the Dissolution Rate of Two Different Brands of Amoxicillin Capsule having Same Dose

Requirements: Volumetric flask, beakers, test tubes, UV spectrophotometer, UV quartz cells, dissolution apparatus I (IP), pipette, funnel, filter paper, amoxicillin tablets of two different brands having same dose.

Reference: Refer any book given in the list of books at the beginning of this manual.

Principle

Capsules are solid dosage form in which drug substance is enclosed within hard or soft soluble shell of gelatin. Dissolution testing for hard gelatin capsules (HGC) is performed using USP apparatus 2. A "sinker" is required to weight the sample of capsule down until it disintegrates and releases its contents at the bottom of the vessel. The sinker has to hold the capsule in a reproducible and stable position directly below the paddle, but it needs to be constructed in such a fashion that it doesn't affect hydrodynamic flow within the vessel nor should it appreciably reduce the surface area of the capsule available to the dissolution medium. Dissolution testing for soft gelatine capsules (SGC), is also performed using USP apparatus 2. For SGC which are dietary supplements, the USP has added a rupture test based on the time needed for capsule shell to rupture in 500 ml water. The capsule shell must rupture within 15 minutes but no drug release is measured.

Amoxicillin is a penicillin antibiotic and is used to treat infections caused by bacteria, such as ear infections, bladder infections, pneumonia, gonorrhea, and E. coli or salmonella infection. Amoxicillin is also sometimes used together with another antibiotic called clarithromycin (Biaxin) to treat stomach ulcers caused by Helicobacter pylori infection. In this experiment two different brands of Amoxicillin capsules having same dose are used for dissolution study in order to find out which brand is superior. Other dissolution conditions are kept similar. The brand which releases the maximum amount of drug in desired period of time is considered superior.

Procedure

Step I: Preparation of calibration curve

1. Accurately weigh 10 mg of drug reference and transfer it into a 100 mL volumetric flask through funnel.

2. Dissolve the drug in distilled water and make up the volume up to 100 mL (stock solution).

3. Take 0.2, 0.4, 0.6, 0.8, 1, 1.2, 1.4, 1.6, 1.8 and 2 mL of stock to the 10 mL volumetric flask separately and make up the volume up to 10 mL with distilled water.

4. Clean the quartz cells by rinsing them with distilled water.

5. Add blank solution (dilution media) to both the cells and do base line correction.

6. Replace the blank solution from one of the cells with drug dilution and carry out the spectrum analysis from 200- 800 nm.

7. Obtain the λ_{max} for the drug and use the wavelength for further absorption readings.

8. Again add blank solution (dilution media) to both the cell and set auto zero at λ_{max} obtained in step 7.

9. Replace the solution from one of the cells with drug dilutions prepared in step 3 and record the absorption readings.

10. Draw a graph between absorption (Y axis) and concentration (X axis) to obtain the calibration curve.

Note: Use methanol or Sodium lauryl sulphate solution as per requirement for solubilization of drug.

Step II: Dissolution study

1. Clean the vessel and place 900 mL of deareated dissolution medium (distilled water or 0.1 N HCl) in the vessel of apparatus I (I.P.) and set temperature at $37 \pm 2\,^{\circ}\text{C}$.

2. Place one tablet in the vessel and operate the rotation of paddle at 50 rpm.

3. Withdraw the 5 mL sample from zone midway between the surface of dissolution medium and the top of the rotating paddle at the defined time intervals (0, 10, 15, 20 30, and 45 min).

4. Add 5 mL of fresh dissolution media at time of each withdrawal.

5. Filter the sample, make the proper dilutions (if needed) and measure the absorbance of samples by using UV spectrophotometer at respective λ_{max}.

6. Calculate concentration of drug using calibration curve.

7. Calculate the cumulative amount of drug released at different points using the following equation.

   Cumulative amount drug released = Concentration (µg/mL) × 900 × Dilution factor / Labeled amount of drug

8. Construct the drug release profile by taking the cumulative amount of drug released on the y-axis and time on the x-axis.

Observations

Table 5.1 Dissolution data of amoxicillin capsule (Brand A)

Time (min)	Absorbance (nm)	Concentration (mg/mL)	Dilution factor	Amount released (mg)
0				
5				
10				
15				
20				
30				
45				

Calculations

Cumulative amount drug released = Concentration (µg/mL) × 900 × Dilution factor / Labeled amount of drug

Table 5.2 Dissolution data of amoxicillin capsule (Brand B)

Time (min)	Absorbance (nm)	Concentration (mg/mL)	Dilution factor	Amount released (mg)
0				
5				
10				
15				
20				
30				
45				

Results: Comparative dissolution profiles of different brands of amoxicillin capsules were studied and brand _________was found better than brand ______as it has given the higher amount drug released.

Precautions

Same as previous experiment.

6

To Compare the Dissolution Profile of Immediate Release and Sustained Release Tablets of Same Drug

Requirements: Volumetric flask, beakers, test tubes, UV spectrophotometer, UV quartz cells, dissolution apparatus I (IP), pipette, funnel, filter paper, amoxicillin tablets of two different brands having same dose.

Reference: Refer any book given in the list of books at the beginning of this manual.

Principle

Dissolution tests have been successfully implemented on conventional dosage forms; there are enormous difficulties in establishing proper dissolution test conditions and parameters for testing sustained or controlled release oral dosage forms because of prolonged gastro-intestinal residence of the dosage form and variability in physiological conditions of the gastrointestinal tract. In an ideal situation, an extended release oral dosage form should be tested *in vitro* throughout the entire physiological pH (1-7.8) of the GI tract in order to simulate the *in vivo* conditions. The physico-chemical and physiological properties of the GI fluid where release of the drug from the administered dosage form occurs are determined by many factors:

(a) the state of the stomach when the dosage form is taken

(b) the nature of food

(c) excipients of the dosage form itself and co-current administration of other drugs.

On an empty stomach an oral dosage form is known to reach the intestine in as little as 10 min whereas in a fed stomach an extended release pellet formulation had gastric emptying times of 119-285 min depending on the size of food administered (light vs. heavy). Another parameter of the dissolution medium which plays a significant role in the dissolution process is its ionic strength. An ideal dissolution apparatus for extended release product should be able to simulate:

(i)   the entire pH range of the GI tract according to the desire of the formulation scientist,

(ii) food induced physiological change that occur in the GI tract, and

(iii) the motility pattern and other mechanical forces encountered by the dosage form in the GI tract.

So once we get dissolution study data for sustained release and immediate release we plot a graph between % release and time, and we get a graph depicting the release pattern. Therefore for immediate release dosage form a simple graph is obtained while for sustained release first a faster release pattern is observed in order to reach the therapeutic range and there after a constant release pattern is observed for the predeter-mined time interval.

Procedure

Step I: Preparation of calibration curve

1. Accurately weigh 10 mg of drug reference and transfer it into a 100 mL volumetric flask through funnel.

2. Dissolve the drug in distilled water and make up the volume up to 100 mL (stock solution).

3. Take 0.2, 0.4, 0.6, 0.8, 1, 1.2, 1.4, 1.6, 1.8 and 2 mL of stock to the 10 mL volumetric flask separately and make up the volume up to 10 mL with distilled water.

4. Clean the quartz cells by rinsing them with distilled water.

5. Add blank solution (dilution media) to both the cells and do base line correction.

6. Replace the blank solution from one of the cells with drug dilution and carry out the spectrum analysis from 200- 800 nm.

7. Obtain the λ_{max} for the drug and use the wavelength for further absorption readings.

8. Again add blank solution (dilution media) to both the cell and set auto zero at λ_{max} obtained in step 7.

9. Replace the solution from one of the cells with drug dilutions prepared in step 3, and record the absorption readings.

10. Draw a graph between absorption (Y axis) and concentration (X axis) to obtain the calibration curve.

Note: Use methanol or Sodium lauryl sulphate solution as per requirement for solubilization of drug.

Step II. Dissolution study

1. Clean the vessel and place 900 mL of deareated dissolution medium (distilled water or 0.1 N HCl) in the vessel of apparatus I (I.P.) and set temperature at $37 \pm 2\,^{\circ}C$.

2. Place one tablet in the vessel and operate the rotation of paddle at 50 rpm.

3. Withdraw the 5 mL sample from zone midway between the surface of dissolution medium and the top of the rotating paddle at the defined time intervals (0, 10, 15, 20 30, and 45 min).

4. Add 5 mL of fresh dissolution media at time of each withdrawal.

5. Filter the sample, make the proper dilutions (if needed) and measure the absorbance of samples by using UV spectrophotometer at respective λ_{max}.

6. Calculate concentration of drug using calibration curve.

7. Calculate the cumulative amount of drug released at different points using the following formula.

Cumulative amount drug released = Concentration (μg/mL) $\times$ 900 $\times$ Dilution factor / Labeled amount of drug

8. Construct the drug release profile by taking the cumulative amount of drug released on the y-axis and time on the x-axis.

Observations

Table 6.1 Dissolution data of amoxicillin tablet (conventional)

Time (min)	Absorbance (nm)	Concentration of diluted solution (mg/mL)	Dilution factor	Amount released (mg)
0				
5				
10				
15				
20				
30				
45				

Calculations

Cumulative amount drug released =   Concentration (μg/mL) $\times$ 900 $\times$ Dilution factor / Labeled amount of drug

Table 6.2 Dissolution data of amoxicillin tablet (Sustain release)

Time (Hrs)	Absorbance (nm)	Concentration of diluted solution (mg/mL)	Dilution factor	Amount released (mg)
0				
0.25				
0.5				
1				
1.5				
2				
2.5				
3				
3.5				
4				
12				
24				

Results: The maximum amount of the drug released was found to be ________ mg in ________ min for the immediate release tablet while the maximum amount of the drug released was found to be ________ mg in ________ min for the sustained release tablet.

Precautions

Same as previous experiment.

PHARMA TRIVIA: SELF EVALUATION TEST

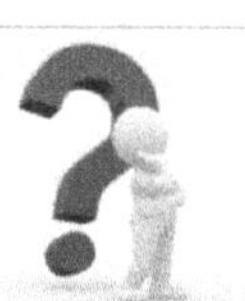

1. Define the term dissolution?

2. Why dissolution testing is used for pharmaceuticals?

3. Write the name of dissolution apparatus for immediate release dosage forms?

4. What are the factors affecting the dissolution rate?

5. Draw dissolution curves for conventional and controlled release tablets?

6. Define the term "biorelevant dissolution media".

7. Explain "sink" and "non-sink" condition for dissolution.

8. Write the Noyes-Whitney's equation for the study of dissolution of drugs.

9. Write the dissolution apparatus classification for different dosage form mentioned in the USP.

10. Write the name of dissolution apparatus for transdermal patches.

3
Tablets

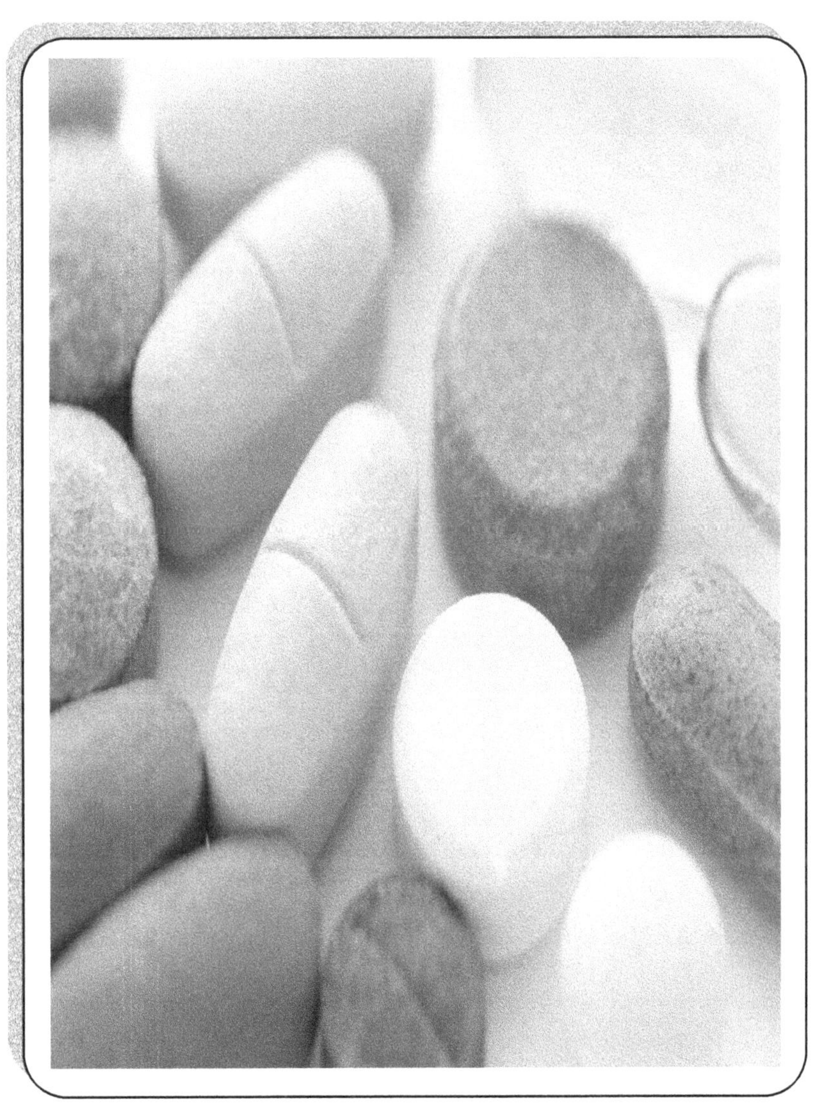

Pharmaceutical tablets are solid flat or biconcave disc unit dosage forms prepared by compressing a drug or a mixture of drugs with or without suitable diluents. They differ in shape as well as in size and weight, depending on the amount of medicinal substances and the intended mode of administration.

Advantages

1. Accurate dose and lees content variability.
2. Lightest and most compact of all oral dosage forms.
3. Convenience and ease of handling and administration.
4. Easiest and cheapest to package and transport.
5. Better suited to large scale production than other unit oral forms.
6. Simplicity and economy in production.
7. Best combined chemical, mechanical and microbiologic stability.
8. Certain special release profile product can be obtained such as enteric or delayed release product.
9. Product identification is simplest and cheapest.
10. Onset of action is fast.

Limitations

1. Some drugs are difficult to compress so as to form tablet.
2. Drugs with bitter taste or objectionable odour and drugs that are sensitive to oxygen or atmospheric moisture are not suitable for tablet dosage form.
3. Drug with poor wetting, slow dissolution properties, relatively large dosages, or combination of these features may not provide sufficient bioavailability of the drug when formulated as tablet.

Types of Tablet

The tablet can be classified on the basis of their method of preparation or route of administration or mechanism of drug release. The detailed classification is given below

1. Molded Tablets

    I. Hypodermic tablets

    II. Dispensing tablets

2. Compressed Tablets

I. Tablets Ingested Orally

(a) Compressed tablets

(b) Multiple compressed tablets

(c) Delayed action and enteric coated tablets

(d) Sugar and chocolate coated tablets

(e) Film coated tablets

(f) Chewable tablets

II. Tablets Used in Oral Cavity

(a) Buccal and subligual tablets

(b) Torches and lozeges

(c) Dental cones

(d) Mouth dissolving tablets

III. Tablets Administered by Other Routes

(a) Implantation tablets

(b) Vaginal tablets

IV. Tablets Used to Prepare Solutions

(a) Effervescent tablets

(b) Dispensing tablets

(c) Hypodermic tablets

(d) Tablet triturates

3. Multiple Compressed Tablets

I. Layered

(a) Tablet within a Tablet

(b) Two Part tablet

(c) Three Layer tablet

II. Compression Coated

Tablet Excipients

In addition to the active or therapeutic ingredients, tablets contain a number of inert materials known as additives or excipients. These are discussed below.

1. **Diluents:** These are the substances which are added to increase the bulk, when the drug dosage itself is inadequate to produce the bulk. When the dose is high no diluents is required.

   Examples: Anhydrous Lactose, Directly Compressible Starches, Cellulose Derivatives, Mannitol, Sorbitol, Dextrose Avicel, Dicalcium Phosphate etc.

2. **Binders:** These are added in liquid or dry form to bind the powder in a coherent mass so that granules can be made. The binders can be sprayed, poured or admixed into the powders to be agglomerated.

   Examples: Acacia, Tragacanth, Gelatin, Starch paste, Polyvinyl pyrrolidone (PVP), Cellulose derivatives etc.

3. **Disintegrants:** These are added to facilitate the break up of tablet when it comes in contact with water or gastrointestinal fluid.

   Examples: Starch, Avicel, Sodium alginates, NaCMC, Gelatin, Bentonite.

   Superdisintegrants: Compounds, which possess exceptional ability to disintegrate tablet as well as relative ease with which they can be processed into tablet formulation, are termed as Superdisintegrants.

   Examples: Ac-Di-sol (crosslinked NaCMC), Explotab (Sodium Starch Glycolate) and Povidon XL (crosslinked polyvinyl pyrrolidone) are few such compounds.

4. **Lubricants:** Reduce the friction between the wall of tablet and die cavity wall during compression and ejection.

   Examples: Water Soluble- PEG (4000, 6000 & 8000), SLS, Sodium Benzoate.

   Water Insoluble- Stearic acid and its salts, Talc, Waxes, Paraffins, Light mineral oils.

5. **Antiadherent:** Reduce sticking of tablet granules or powder to punch and also to the die wall.

   Examples: Starch, Talc, metallic stearates (magnesium stearate) colloidal silica (Cab-O –Sil, syloid).

6. **Glidants:** Improve the flow of materials from hopper into die cavity.

   Examples: Starch, Silica derivatives, Talc, Pyrogenic silica (Aerosil/ Cab-O-Sil) etc.

7. **Organoleptic additives:** These include colouring, flavouring and sweetening agents.

   Coloring agent: Soluble dyes, Insoluble pigments, and Lakes.

   Examples: Synthetic- FD & C colours.

   Natural- Red (Beet, Cochineal), Purple (Grape skin extract), Yellow (Turmeric, Riboflavin), Orange (saffron)

   Flavoring agent: Spray dried and other flavors.

   Sweeteners: Natural -Mannnitol, Sucrose, Dextrose

   Artificial: Saccharine and Aspartame

Method of Preparation

1. Granulation Compression Method
   (a) Wet granulation
   (b) Dry granulation

2. Direct compression

Evaluation

Evaluation of tablet is divided into two categories

1. **Non-official:** General appearance, Organoleptic Properties, Size, Shape, Thickness

2. **Official:** Disintegration, Weight variation, Content uniformity, Dissolution, Friability.

7

To Study the Flow Properties of Various Drugs and Excipients used in Tablet Manufacturing

Requirements: Equipment: Funnel, stand, butter paper, ruler, measuring cylinder, weighing balance, drugs (aspirin, paracetamol, sulfasalazine, ascorbic acid), excipients (lactose, mannitol, starch, MCC, magnesium stearate, talc, stearic acid etc.)

Reference: Refer any book given in the list of books at the beginning of this manual.

Principle

The flow properties of solids have great impact on the tableting and encapsulation processes as their manufacturing require the flow of powder materials from a storage container to filling stations, such as tablet dies or capsule fillers. Weight uniformity also depends on uniform and rapid flow of powders. The flow properties of solids also have great influence on the mixing and demixing of powders that take place before tableting or encapsulation. Different flow properties are required at different stages of processing and should be carefully taken into consideration during formulation and process validation. Particle size of excipients has a significant effect on the content uniformity since as the particle sizes of excipients increase, the degree of mixing decreases. Pharmaceutical powders can be either cohesive or free flowing. The various factors influencing the flow of solids are:

(a) Nature of Powders and Granulations: Some powders have good flowability to flow into the tablet compression die whereas some others are made into granules to improve flowability.

(b) Particle Size and Size Distribution: larger particle flow faster than smaller particles (fine particles are more cohesive than coarser particles which are influenced more by gravitational forces)

(c) Shape Factors and Surface Morphology: Flowability of powders decreases as the shapes of particles become more irregular.

(d) Moisture and Static Charge: Very low moisture can hinder flow since powder are likely to develop electrostatic charge.

(e) Effects of Temperature: The cohesion of powder decrease as the temperature is decreased.

Characterization of Powder Flow

A) Indirect Methods:

    I. By angle of repose: Maximum angle obtained between surface of powder heap and horizontal plane. It measures resistant to particle movement.

$$\tan\theta = \text{Height of heap (h) / Radius of Heap (r)}$$

Therefore

$$\theta = \tan^{-1} h/r$$

Table 7.1 Relation between angle of repose (θ) and type of flow

S. No.	Angle of Repose ($^\circ$)	Type of Flow
1.	< 25	Excellent
2.	25-30	Good
3.	30- 40	Satisfactory
4.	40-50	Poor
5.	> 50	Very Poor

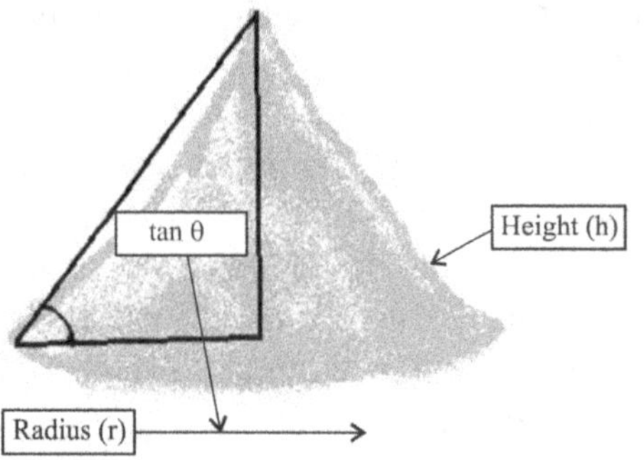

Fig. 7.1 Angle of repose.

II. By Bulk density measurements:

1. Carr's index: Indication of ease with which a material can be induced to flow. This parameter is calculated by following formula:

> **Carr's index =**
> **(Tap density – Bulk density)/Tap density × 100**

Table 7.2 Relation between CCI and type of flow

S. No.	Comressibility Index (CCI)	Type of Flow
1.	5-15	Excellent
2.	12-16	Good
3.	18-21	Fair
4.	> 23	Poor flow

2. Hausner's ratio: This is related to interparticle friction and calculated by following formula.

> **Hausner's ratio = Tap density/Bulk density**

Table 7.3 Relationship between hausner ratio and type of flow

S. No.	Hausner's Ratio	Type of Flow
1.	1.02 – 1.14	Excellent
2.	1.14 – 1.20	Good
3.	1.20 – 1.30	Satisfactory
4.	1.30 – 1.51	Poor
5.	1.51 - 1.6	Very Poor
6.	> 1.6	Extremely Poor

B) Direct Methods:

1. Hopper flow rate: measure the rate at which powder discharges from a hopper.

2. Recording flow meter: powder is allowed to discharge from a hopper or container   on to a balance.

Powder flow can be improved by following methods

1. Alteration of particle size and size distribution

2. Alteration of particle shape

3. Alteration of surface forces

4. Use of flow activators

Procedure

1. Bulk Density Measurement

Method

1. Take a dry and clean measuring cylinder.

2. Weigh 25 grams of sample (drugs or excipients) and place carefully into the measuring cylinder.

3. Note down the volume occupied by the sample (drugs or excipients). Repeat this experiment three times.

4. Calculate bulk density by the following formula.

Bulk Density (BD) = Weight of the sample (drugs or excipients)/ Volume of the sample (drugs or excipients)

Observations

Table 7.4 Bulk density of drug or excipients

S. No.	Weight of Powder (gm)	Volume of powder (ml)	Bulk density (gm/ml)	Average Bulk Density (gm/ml)
1				
2				
3				

2. Tapped Density Measurement

Method

1. Place graduated cylinder containing the 25 gm of powder on the bulk density equipment and tap manually or mechanically until constant volume is obtained.

2. Stop tapping and note down the final volume.

3. Repeat this experiment three times and calculate average tapped density

4. Calculate the Tapped Density by the following formula.

Tapped Density (TD) = Weight of the sample (drugs and excipients)/Tapped volume of the sample (drugs or excipients)

Observations

Table 7.5 Tapped density of drug/excipients

S. No.	Weight of Powder (gm)	Tapped Volume of powder (ml)	Tapped density (gm/ml)	Average Tapped Density (gm/ml)
1				
2				
3				

Note: For the determination of tap density 'Tap density apparatus (USP)' is used at industrial level.

3. Hausner's Ratio

Calculate by following formula

$$\textbf{Hausner's Ratio} = \frac{TD}{BD}$$

where, TD – Tapped density

    BD – Bulk density

Compare the value with value given in the Table 7.3 and mark the flow accordingly

4. Carr's Compressibility Index (CCI)

Calculate by using following formula:

$$\textbf{\% Compressibility} = \frac{TD - BD}{TD} \times 100$$

where, TD – Tapped density and BD – Bulk density

Compare the calculated value with a value given in Table 7.2 and mark the flow accordingly

5. Angle of Repose

It is defined as the maximum angle that can be obtained between the free standing surface of a powder heap and the horizontal plane.

Method

1. Set a funnel at a height of 4 cm from base on a stand.
2. Take approximately 10 gms of sample (drugs and excipients).
3. Allow them to fall through a funnel over a clean weighing paper on a horizontal plane. Continue adding the sample (drugs and

excipients) till the excess of sample (drugs and excipients) slide down the sides of the heap formed.

4. Measure the critical height of the heap and radius of the base of the heap of powder

5. Calculate by following formula

$$\theta = \tan^{-1} h/r$$

where, $\theta \rightarrow$ Angle of repose.

   $h \rightarrow$ height of the heap of powder

   $r \rightarrow$ radius of the base of the heap of powder

6. Repeat this experiment three times and calculate average angle of repose.

7. Compare the calculated value with value given in the Table 7.1 and mark the flow accordingly

Results:

- The flow properties of various drugs & excipients were studied.

- The results are compiled and shown in table given below.

S. No.	Powder	Carr's Compressibility Index	Hausner's Ratio	Angle of Repose	Inference
1.	Drug 1				
2.	Drug 2				
3.	Drug 3				
4.	Drug 4				
5.	Excipient 1				
6.	Excipient 2				
7.	Excipient 3				
8.	Excipient 4				

8

To Study the Structure and Functioning of Various Types of Tablet Compression Machines

Requirements: Single punch machine, rotary compression machine.

Reference: Refer any book given in the list of books at the beginning of this manual.

Principle

All tableting machines employ the same basic principle-they compress the granular or powdered mixture of ingredients in a die between two punches which are of same set and are called a "station of tooling".

Types of Tablet Compression Machines

Tablet machines can be divided into two distinct categories as per station of tooling (Fig. 8.1a & b).

(i) Those with a single set of tooling- "single station' or "single-punch" or "eccentric" compression machine.

(ii) Those with several stations of tooling- "multi-station" or "rotary" compression machine.

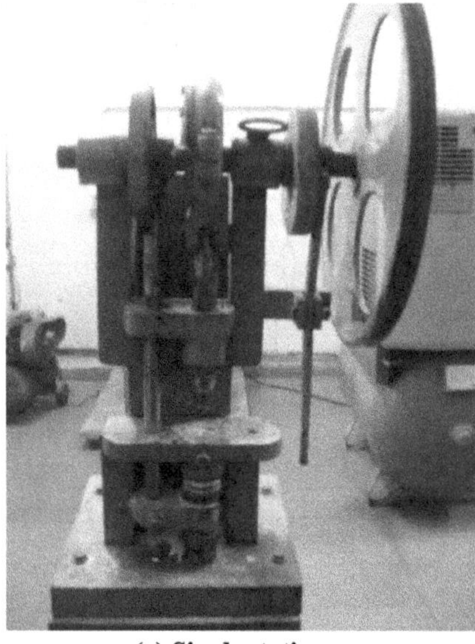

(a) Single station

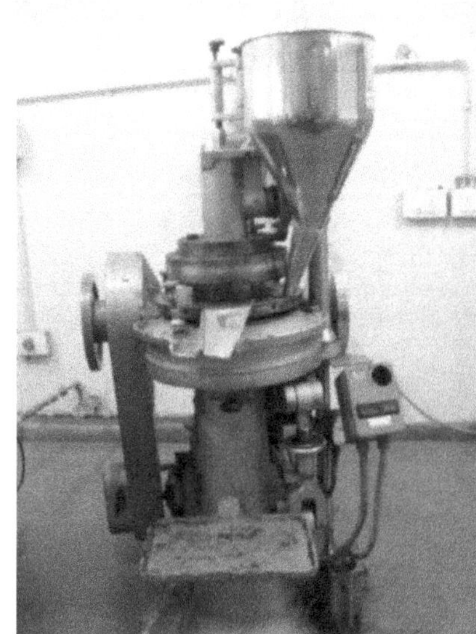

(b) Multi station

Fig. 8.1 Tablet press.

Structure of Tablet Compression Machine

All the tablet compression machines are designed with the following basic components:

A. Hopper(s) for holding and feeding granules/powder for compression

B. Feeding tray

C. Dies that defines the size and shape of the tablet

D. Punches for compression of granules/powders within the dies

E. Cam tracks for guiding the movement of the punches

- **Hopper(s)** – hopper is a cone shaped stainless steel vessel to hold granules (Fig. 8.2). It supplies the granules to the feeding tray. Number of hoppers can be added as per need of the amount of granules in die punches.

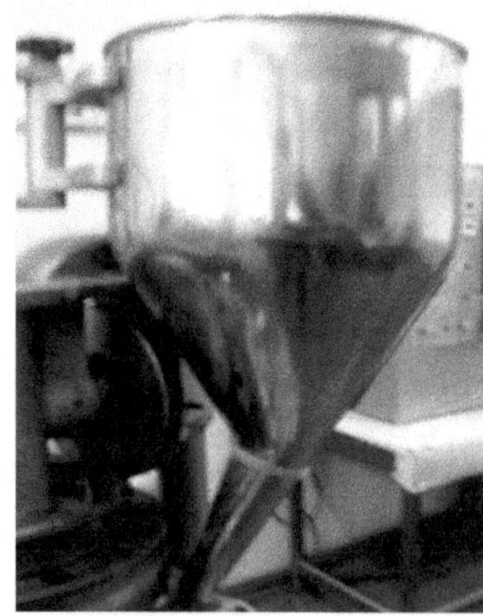

Fig. 8.2 Hopper.

- **Feeding tray** – granules from the hopper empties into feed frame or feeding tray, which has several interconnected compartments (Fig 8.3). These compartments spread the granules over the wide area to provide time for the dies to fill. A scrapper is attached at the end of the feed tray, which detaches the tablet from the machine on ejection.

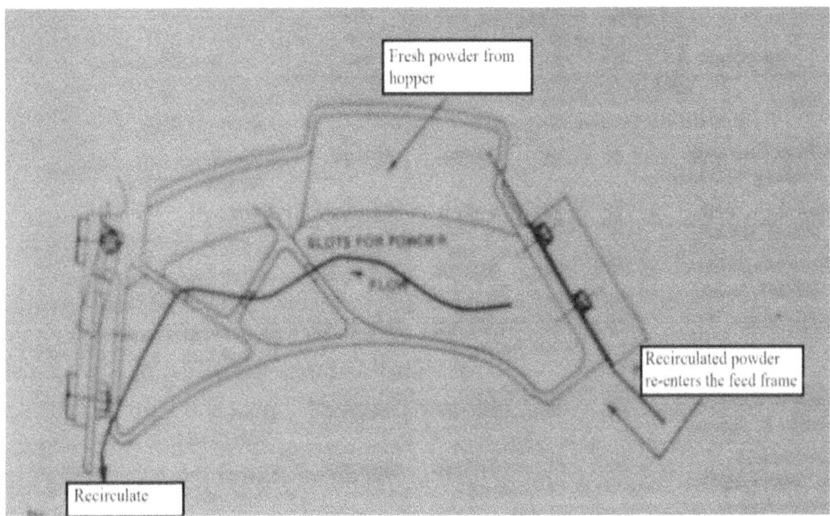

Fig. 8.3 Feed frame and parts.

- **Dies** – The tablet assumes the shape and size of punches and dies used. While round tablets are used most commonly for tablet compression, other shapes like oval, square, triangular, hexagonal etc., are also being used. Dies come in set with the punches and are made up of stainless steel (Fig. 8.4).

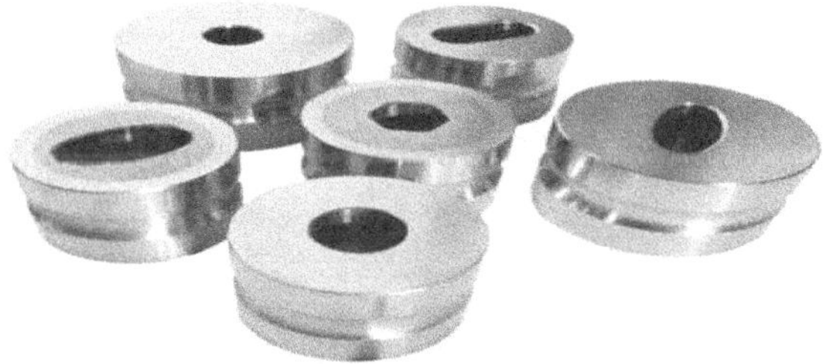

Fig. 8.4 Dies for tablet compression.

- **Punches** – punches are a set of rod like structure made to press the granules inside cavity with great force to make tablets (Fig. 8.5). Each punch set contains a two identical length punches (upper punch and lower punch). However the neck of the lower punch is longer than that of upper punch. Punches are of various sizes and shapes as per requirement. Some of them are plane surfaced while others are embossed with trademarks or scoring line (mark for breaking tablet).

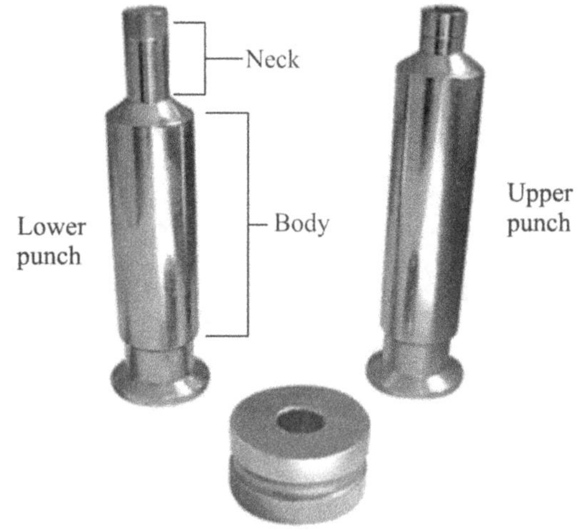

Fig. 8.5 Tablet compression punch set.

- **Cam tracks** – Cam tracks are the paths which guides punches at different stages of tablet compression (Fig. 8.6). They make the punches to come closer on compression stage and then move apart. Also they guide lower punch to move to die level for the ejection of the tablet.

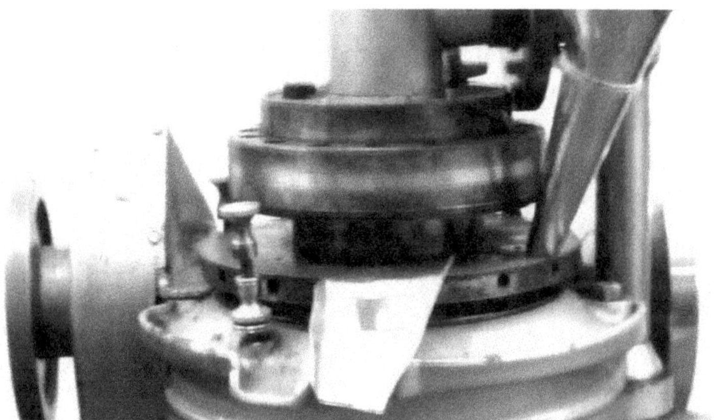

Fig. 8.6 Cam- tracks.

Working of Tablet Compression Machines

A. Single station tablet compression machines

Single station machines are the simplest tablet compression machines. They have only one set of die-punch set and are often operated manually or attached with a driving motor.

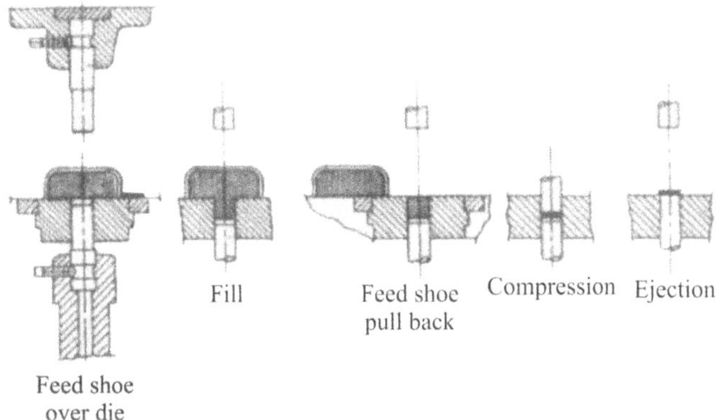

Fig. 8.7 Various stages of tablet compression in a single station tableting press.

The granules ready for compression are placed in the hopper of the machine from where it feeds into the die by feed shoe (Fig. 8.7), where it is compressed in between two punches (upper and lower punch).

The lower punch is adjusted inside die in such a way that it makes sufficient space to be filled by granules. This stage is called filling. In the next stage feed shoe pulls back the excess of material and upper punch is lowered to compress the granules in the cavity into tablets. The pressure required for the compression is adjusted from the upper punch. In the ejection stage the upper punch is raised and lower punch is also rise in die cavity to its upper level to eject the tablet, which is then removed by the scrapper.

B. Multi-station (rotary) tablet compression machine:

For increased production, rotary machines offer great advantages. A head carry a number of punches and dies revolves continuously while the tablet granules runs from the hopper, through a feed frame and into the dies placed in a large, steel plate revolving under it (Fig. 8.8). This method promotes a uniform fill of the die and therefore an accurate weight for the tablets.

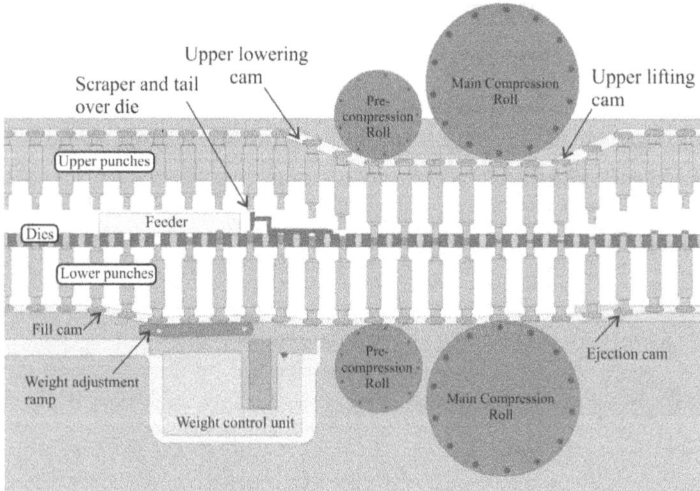

Fig. 8.8 Various stages of tablet compression in a multi-station tableting press.

Compression takes place as the upper and lower punches pass between a pair of rollers. This action produces a slow squeezing effect on the material in the die cavity from the top and bottom and so gives a chance for the entrapped air to escape. The lower punch lifts up and ejects the tablet at the ejection stage. Tablet is then removed by the scrapper attached to feed frame and collected. The excess of material re-enter the feed frame and even filled to the die cavity. The process moves on continuously producing large number of tablets in small period of time.

Results: Different types of tablet machine and their parts were studied.

9

To Evaluate Different Types of Tablet

Requirements: Glass apparatus, measuring cylinders, weighing balance, dissolution apparatus, disintegration apparatus, vernier calliper, scale, hardness tester, friability tester, UV-spectrophotometer, various types of tablets.

Reference: Refer any book given in the list of books at the beginning of this manual.

Principle

Official Standards as per I.P./B.P./U.S.P.

Table 9.1 Comparison of different pharmacopoeial quality control tests

Pharmacopoeias	Type of tablet	Tests to be performed
British Pharmacopoeia (2008)	For all tablets	a. Content of active ingredients b. Disintegration c. Uniformity of content d. Labeling
	Uncoated tablet	a. Disintegration test b. Uniformity of weight
	Effervescent tablet	a. Disintegration test b. Uniformity of weight
	Coated tablet	a. Disintegration test b. Uniformity of weight
	Gastro resistant tablet	a. Disintegration test
	Modified release tablet	a. Uniformity of weight
	Tablet for use in mouth	a. Uniformity of weight

Table 9.1 *Contd...*

Pharmacopoeias	Type of tablet	Tests to be performed
	Soluble tablet	a. Disintegration test
		b. Uniformity of weight
	Dispersible tablet	a. Disintegration test
		b. Uniformity of dispersion
		c. Uniformity of weight
INDIAN PHARMACOPOEIA (2010)	Uncoated tablet	a. Uniformity of container content
		b. Content of active ingredient
		c. Uniformity of weight
		d. Uniformity of content
		e. Disintegration test
	Enteric coated tablet	a. Disintegration test
	Dispersible tablet	a. Uniformity of dispersion
		b. Disintegration
	Soluble tablet	a. Disintegration test
	Effervescent tablet	b. Disintegration/ Dissolution / Dispersion test

I. Compendial Tests

1. Content of active ingredient

- Determine the amount of active ingredient(s) by method described in the assay (IP, BP or USP) and calculate the amount of active ingredient(s) in each tablet.
- The range lies within the range for the content of active ingredient(s) stated in the official monograph.
- This range is based on the requirement that 20 tablets, or such other numbers as may be indicated in the monograph, are used in the assay. Where 20 tablets cannot be obtained, a smaller number, which must not be less than 5, may be used, but to allow for sampling errors the tolerances are widened in accordance to Table 9.2.
- The requirements of the table apply when the stated limits are between 90 and 100%.
- For limits other than 90 to 100%, proportionately smaller or larger allowances should be made.

Table 9.2 Tolerance limits for the content uniformity

Weight of active ingredients in each tablet	Subtract from lower limit for samples of (g)			Add to the upper limit for samples of			Number of tablets
	15	**10**	**5**	**15**	**10**	**5**	
0.12 g or less	0.2	0.7	1.6	0.3	0.8	1.8	
More than 0.12 g but less than 0.3 g	0.2	0.5	1.2	0.3	0.6	1.5	
0.3 g or more	0.1	0.2	0.8	0.2	0.4	1.0	

Observation

Table 9.3 Active ingredient in tablet

Type of Tablet	Active ingredient in 20 tablets (mg)	Active ingredient in 1 tablet (mg)
Uncoated tablet		
Film coated tablet		
Enteric Coated Tablet		
Sugar coated tablet		
Sustain Release Tablet		
Effervescent Tablet		
Chewable Tablet		
Soluble/ Dispersible Tablet		
Fast Dissolving Tablet		

2. Uniformity of weight/Weight variation test

This test is not applicable to coated tablets (Sugar and enteric coated tablet) except film-coated tablets. The test is also not applicable to the tablets which are required to comply with the test for 'uniformity of content' for all active ingredients.

- Weigh 20 tablets selected at random and calculate the average weight.

- Weigh the individual tablets separately.

- Not more than 2 of the individual weights deviate from the average weight by more than percentage shown in Table 9.5 and none deviates by more than twice that percentage.

Table 9.4 Permitted weight variation

Pharmacopoeia	Average Tablet weight (mg)	Maximum % Difference allowed
Indian Pharmacopoeia (I.P.)	≤ 80	±10
	80-250	±7.5
	> 250	±5
United States Pharmacopoeia (U.S.P.)	≤130	±10
	130-324	±7.5
	>324	±5

Example

Weight of 20 tablets (W) = W gm

Average weight of tablet (W/20) = A gm

Suppose A = 100 mg (average weight)

Then according to U.S.P., if A < 130, ± 10% (L) variation is permissible.

Absolute limit of permissible variation (B) = A × L /100

$$= 100 \times 10/100$$
$$= 10 \text{ mg}$$

Then upper limit   =   A + B = C mg (110 mg)

Lower limit   =   A – B = C mg (90 mg)

Therefore, tablets should fall between 110 mg to 90 mg individually. (This example is based on U.S.P. limit)

Table 9.5 Weight variation of tablet

S. No.	Wt of individual tablet (mg)	Inference (Passed/failed)	S. No.	Wt of tablet (mg)	Inference (Pass/fail)
1.	93		11.	108	
2.	95		12.	110	
3.	100		13.	105	
4.	105		14.	100	
5.	95		15.	100	
6.	95		16.	90	
7.	98		17.	85	
8.	95		18.	90	
9.	100		19.	115	
10.	105		20.	90	

Note: The tablet passes the U.S.P. test if not more than 2 tablets are out of the percentage limit allowed. It may be seen from the above table that since number of tablets crossing the limit is not exceeding 2, the hypothetical batch passes the test of weight variation.

Table 9.6 Weight variation of different types of tablets

Weight of Tablets

	Uncoated Tablet	Film Coated Tablet	Enteric Coated Tablet	Sugar Coated Tablet	Sustain Release Tablet	Effervescent Tablet	Chewable Tablet	Soluble/Dispersible Tablet	Fast Dissolving Tablet
1									
2									
3									
4									
5									
6									
7									
8									
9									
10									
11									
12									
13									
14									
15									
16									
17									
18									
19									
20									
Avg Wt.									
Permissible Limit									
Inference									

3. Uniformity of content

This test is applicable to tablets that contain 10 mg or less than 10% w/w of active ingredients. For tablets containing more than one active ingredient carry out the test for each active ingredient that corresponds to aforementioned conditions.

The test for 'Uniformity of content' should be carried out only after the content of active ingredient(s) in a pooled sample of tablets has been shown to be accepted limits of stated limits of the stated content.

- Determine the content of active ingredient(s) in each of the 10 tablets taken at random using the method given in the monograph or by any other suitable analytical method.

- The tablets comply with the test if not more than one of the individual values thus obtained is outside the limits 85 to 115% of the average value and none is outside the limits 75 to 125% of the avg. value.

- If two or three of the individual values are outside the limits 85 to 115% of the average value and none is outside the limits 75 to 125%, repeat the test using another 20 tablets.

- The tablets comply with the test if in the total sample of 30 tablets not more than three of the individual values are outside the limits 85 to 115% and none is outside the limits 75 to 125% of the avg. value.

4. Uniformity of container content

- Select a sample of 10 containers and count the number of tablets in each container.

- The average no. of the contents in the 10 containers is not less than the labelled amount and the no. in any single container is not less than 98% and not more than 102% of the labelled amount.

- If the requirement is not met, count the no. of contents in each of 10 additional containers.

- The average no. in the 20 containers is not less than labelled amount, and the no. in not more than 1 of the 20 containers is less than 98% or more than 102% of the labelled amount.

Observation

Table 9.7 Drug content of different types of tablets

	Drug Content (mg)								
	Uncoated Tablet	Film Coated Tablet	Enteric Coated Tablet	Sugar Coated Tablet	Sustain Release Tablet	Effervescent Tablet	Chewable Tablet	Soluble/ Dispersible Tablet	Fast Dissolving Tablet
1									
2									
3									
4									
5									
6									
7									
8									
9									
10									
Avg. Content									
Range									
Inf.									

Observation

Table 9.8 Container content of different types of tablets

				Container Content					
	Uncoated Tablet	Film Coated Tablet	Enteric Coated Tablet	Sugar Coated Tablet	Sustain Release Tablet	Effervescent Tablet	Chewable Tablet	Soluble/ Dispersible Tablet	Fast Dissolving Tablet
1									
2									
3									
4									
5									
6									
7									
8									
9									
10									
Avg.									
Range									
Inf.									

5. Disintegration test

This test is not applicable to modified-release tablets and tablets for use in mouth. For those tablets for which the 'dissolution test' is included in the individual monograph, the test for disintegration is not required.   While, for the dispersible tablets the test is not performed in disintegration apparatus.

- Switch on the disintegration apparatus and observe the number of strokes (it should be between 28 – 32/min)
- Fill the beaker with 900 ml of specified media, maintain the temperature at 37 ± 2°C.
- Unless otherwise stated in the individual monograph, introduce one tablet into each tube and if directed in the appropriate general monograph, add a disc to each tube.
- Suspend the assembly in the beaker containing the specified liquid and operate the apparatus.
- Record the time at which no particulate material is left on the screen of each test tube.
- Remove the assembly from the liquid.
- The tablets pass the test if all of them have disintegrated.
- If 1or 2 tablets fail to disintegrate, repeat the test on additional 12 tablets; not less than 16 of the total of 18 tablets tested disintegrate.
- If the tablets adhere to the disc and the preparation being examined fails to comply, repeat the test omitting the discs.
- The preparation complies with the test if all the tablets in the repeat test disintegrate.

Table 9.9 Conditions and time for disintegration of various types of tablets

Type of tablet	Medium	Disintegration time	Temp.
Uncoated tablets	Water	Not more than 15 mins.	37 ± 2°C
Coated tablets	Water	Not more than 30 minutes for film-coated tablets and not more than 60 minutes for other coated tablets	37 ± 2°C
Enteric-coated tablets	0.1M HCl (for initial 120 mninutes) and mixed phosphate buffer pH 6.8 (for further 60 minutes)	120 mins. + 60 mins. = 180 mins.	37 ± 2°C
Dispersible and Soluble tablets	Water	≤ 3 minutes	Room temperature 24°C to 26°C
Effervescent tablets	Water (250 ml) in a beaker	≤ 5 minutes	Room temperature

Observation

Table 9.10 Disintegration time of various tablets

	Disintegration Time								
	Uncoated Tablet	Film Coated Tablet	Enteric Coated Tablet	Sugar Coated Tablet	Sustain Release Tablet	Effervescent Tablet	Chewable Tablet	Soluble/ Dispersible Tablet	Fast Dissolving Tablet
1									
2									
3									
4									
5									
6									
Avg									
Inf.									

6. Uniformity of dispersion (For Dispersible tablets)

This test is applicable only to dispersible tablets.

Method

- Place 2 tablets in 100 ml of water and stir gently until completely dispersed.

- A smooth dispersion is obtained which passes through a sieve screen with a normal mesh aperture of 710 um (sieve no. 22) without any remains of the dispersed tablet.

7. Dissolution

Refer the "dissolution experiments" (experiment no. 3. page no. 22).

II. Non-compendial Tests

There are number of tests frequently applied to the tablets (non-compendial) as a part of a manufacturer's own product specification. Details of these tests are given below:

1. General appearance

Visually inspect the tablets for the following characteristics:

- Size (Vernier caliper)
- Shape
- Thickness (Vernier caliper)
- Colour
- Odour
- Taste
- Surface textures

Observation

Table 9.11 General appearance

		Uncoated Tablet	Film Coated Tablet	Enteric Coated Tablet	Sugar Coated Tablet	Sustain Release Tablet	Effervescent Tablet	Chewable Tablet	Soluble/ Dispersible Tablet	Fast Dissolving Tablet
Size	1									
	2									
	3									
	4									
	5									
	Avg									
Shape										
Thickness	1									
	2									
	3									
	4									
	5									
	Avg									
Colour										
Odour										
Taste										
Surface Texture										

2. Mechanical strength of tablets

The mechanical properties of pharmaceutical tablets are quantifiable by the

(a) Friability (Official in USP)

(b) Hardness or crushing strength

(a) Friability (Official in USP)

- 10 tablets are weighed and placed in the apparatus where they are exposed to rolling and repeated shocks as they fall 6 inches in each turn within the apparatus.

- After four minutes of this treatment or 100 revolutions, the tablets are weighed and the weight compared with the initial weight.

- The loss due to abrasion is a measure of the tablet friability, using following formula:

$$\boxed{\% \text{ Friability} = (w_0 - w)/w_0 \times 100}$$

where w_0 = Original weight of 20 tablets

   w = Weight of tablets after 100 revolutions

Acceptable limit of friability = upto 1 %

If friability is more than this limit, batch does not pass this test. In case capping is observed, the batch is not suitable for commercial use even if % friability is within limit.

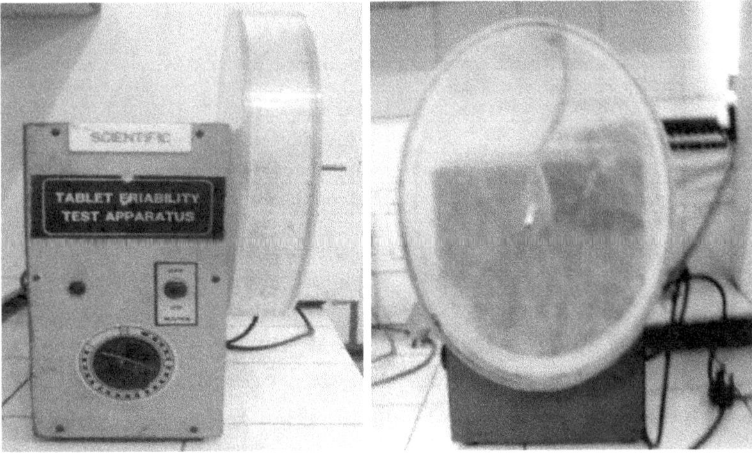

Fig. 9.1 Friability tester.

Observations

Table 9.12 %Friability of different types of tablets

Type of Tablet	Percentage Friability	Inference (passed/failed)
Uncoated tablet		
Film Coated Tablet		
Enteric Coated Tablet		
Sugar Coated Tablet		
Sustain Release Tablet		
Effervescent Tablet		
Chewable Tablet		
Soluble/ Dispersible Tablet		
Fast Dissolving Tablet		

(b) Hardness or crushing strength

The resistance of tablets to capping, abrasion or breakage under conditions of storage, transportation and handling before usage depends on its hardness. Use Monsanto type, to measures the diametrically applied force required to break the tablet.

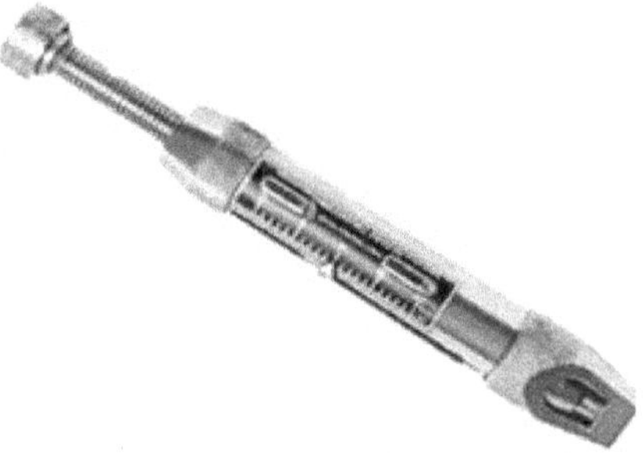

Fig. 9.2 Monsanto hardness tester.

Table 9.13 Hardness limits for various types of tablets

S. No.	Type of tablet	Hardness
1.	Oral tablets	5 to 10 kg/cm^2
2.	Hypodermic and chewable tablet	3 kg/cm^2
3.	Sustained release tablets	10 to 20 kg/cm^2

Note: Limits can vary according to the size and the shapes of the tablets.

Method

- Take one tablet and put it diametrically between the jaws of Monsanto hardness tester. Adjust zero on scale.
- Apply force and note down the breaking point of the tablet.
- Repeat experiment for another two tablets.

Observations

Table 9.14 Hardness of tablets

S. No.	No. of tablets	Hardness (kg/cm^2)	Avg. hardness (kg/cm^2)	Inference (passed/ failed)
1	1			
2	2			
3	3			

Table 9.15 Hardness of various types of tablets

S. No.	Type of Tablet	Average Hardness (Kg/cm^2)
1.	Uncoated tablet	
2.	Film coated tablet	
3.	Enteric coated tablet	
4.	Sugar coated tablet	
5.	Sustain release Tablet	
6.	Effervescent tablet	
7.	Chewable tablet	
8.	Soluble/ dispersible tablet	
9.	Fast dissolving tablet	

Results: The results of various tests are compiled in the table given below:

Type of Tablet	Content of active ingredient (mg)	Uniformity of weight (mg)	Uniformity of content (mg)	Uniformity of container content	Disintegration Time (min)	Friability (%)	Hardness (Kg/cm^2)	Thickness (mm)
Uncoated tablet								
Film Coated Tablet								
Enteric Coated Tablet								
Sugar Coated Tablet								
Sustain Release Tablet								
Effervescent Tablet								
Chewable Tablet								
Soluble/ Dispersible Tablet								
Fast Dissolving Tablet								

10

To Prepare and Evaluate Ascorbic Acid/ Aspirin/Paracetamol Granules

Requirements: Excipients, pestle mortar, sieves (#10, 20, & 40), funnel, measuring cylinder, stand.

Reference: Refer any book given in the list of books at the beginning of this manual.

Formula

S. No.	Ingredients	Quantity per tablet	Quantity taken for 30 tablets
1.	Ascorbic acid[*]	50 mg	
2.	Lactose	19 mg	
3.	Starch	15 mg	
4.	Ethyl cellulose	10 mg	
5.	Talc	5 mg	
6.	Magnesium stearate	1 mg	

* In place of ascorbic acid , Aspirin or Paracetamol can be used

Principle

Granulation is the process in which primary powder particles are made to adhere to form larger, multiparticle entities called granules. Granulation is often followed by sieving to get monodispersed granules (similar size range).

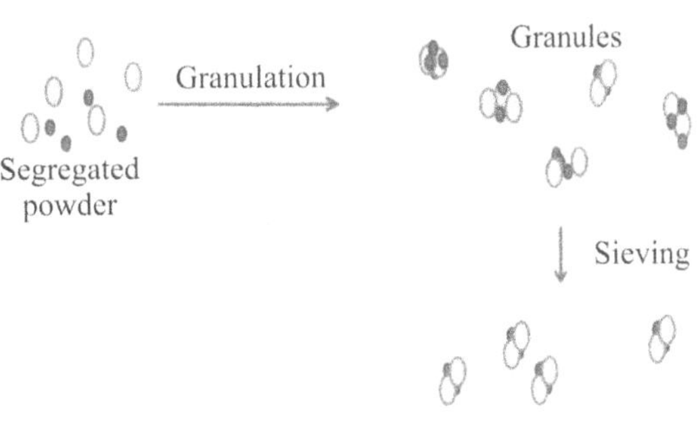

Fig. 10.1 Granulation technique.

Granulation of powdered material provides a number of advantages in pharmaceutical formulations such as:

Need for granulation - The main reasons for granulation are:

1. to improve the flow of powders.
2. to increase the primary particle size by agglomeration.
3. to improve the compression characteristics, which are interdependent on the flow ability of powders
4. to decrease the bulk volume and hence making transportation and storage easier.
5. to reduce dust/environmental hazards,
6. to make powders easier to handle.

Other important applications could be

(i)   provide densification

(ii)   prevent segregation

(iii) improve appearance of material by enhancing better distribution of color and soluble drugs it added to binder solution.

(iv)   To make hydrophobic surfaces more hydrophilic through the addition of surfactants and other water-soluble binders and polymers.

In the present experiment, granules are prepared by non-aqueous wet granulation technique to reduce the degradation of ascorbic acid. Similar strategy can be used with aspirin to avoid the hydrolytic decomposition. Granulation imparts some ideal properties to the formulation excipients during tableting such as good flow and compressibility or they can be directly dispensed in capsules. In the given formula lactose was used as an diluent, starch was used as a disintegrant, ethyl cellulose as binder and talc and magnesium stearate as anti-adherent and glident.

Procedure

- Weigh separately desired quantity of ascorbic acid, lactose, ethyl cellulose and starch. Transfer it to mortar.
- Add ethyl alcohol (non-aqueous granulating solvent) gradually to the above mixture to form soft and non-sticky dough.
- Pass the dough through sieve no. 10 and completely dry granules in an oven at 60 °C.

- Pass the granules through sieve No. 20 superimposed on sieve No. 40.
- Weigh the granules, which pass through sieve No. 20 and are retained on sieve No. 40.
- Add 10% fines (which pass through sieve No. 40) to weighed granules (obtained in previous step).
- Evaluate the granules for various flow properties **(Without glidant).**
- Add talc or magnesium stearate to the granules and mix properly.
- Subject the granules to evaluation tests again **(with glidant).**

Evaluation of Granules: (With and without glidant): Same as experiment number 7.

Results: The results are summarized in following table

S. No.	Parameters	Value without Glidant	Value with Glidant	Inference
1.	Bulk density (gm/cm^3)			
2.	Tapped density (gm/cm^3)			
3.	Hausner's ratio			
4.	Carr's compressibility index			
5.	Angle of repose			

11

To Prepare and Evaluate Effervescent Aspirin Tablets I.P. by Non-Aqueous Wet Granulation Method

Requirements: Pestle mortar, sieves (# 8, 20, 44), filter paper sheets, hardness tester, friabilator, disintegration apparatus.

Reference: Refer any book given in the list of books at the beginning of this manual.

Formula: For 500 mg tablet.

S. No.	Ingredients	Quantity per tablet	Quantity taken for 30 tablets
1.	Acetyl salicylic acid	300 mg	
2.	Lactose	14.5 mg	
3.	Saccharin sodium	2.5 mg	
4.	Citric acid	30 mg	
5.	Calcium carbonate	100 mg	
6.	Ethyl cellulose	15 mg	
7.	Starch	20 mg	
8.	Talc	15 mg	
9.	Magnesium stearate	2.5 mg	

Principle

Non-aqueous wet granulation technique was used in the present experiment for making aspirin tablet to avoid hydrolytic decomposition of aspirin. Wet granulation is the most common technique for tabletting as the granules prepared with this method have all the ideal characteristics.

Advantages of wet granulation method:

- Granules with good flow properties.
- Tablets prepared have good hardness.
- Very efficient mixing of tablet excipients.
- Better binding of tablet excipients.

Disadvantages of wet granulation method:

- Large number of preparation steps.
- High cost.
- Wastage of material.

Wet granulation technique consists of following steps:

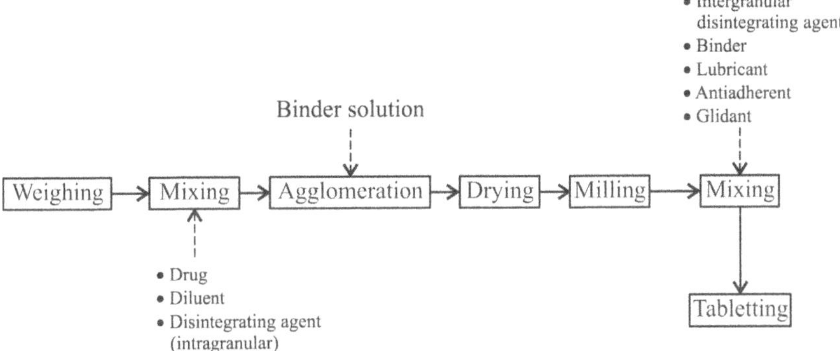

Fig. 11.1 Unit operations in wet granulation tabletting method.

Citric acid and calcium carbonate are included in the formula to provide the effervescence for disintegration. Effervescence leads to faster disintegration of the tablet and the release of the active content.

$$2C_6H_8O_7 + 3CaCO_3 = Ca_3(C_6H_5O_7)_2 + 3CO_2 + 3H_2O$$

Ethyl cellulose is used as binder, lactose as diluents and talc and magnesium stearate as lubricants. Sacchrin sodium is used to mask the bitterness.

Procedure

- Weigh separately desired quantity of aspirin, citric acid, lactose, calcium carbonate, ethyl cellulose, saccharin sodium and starch (first take half quantity of starch). Transfer it to mortar.

- Add ethyl alcohol (non-aqueous granulating solvent) gradually to the above mixture to form soft and non-sticky dough.
- Pass the dough through sieve no. 10 and completely dry granules in an oven at 60 °C.
- Pass the granules through sieve No. 20 superimposed on sieve No. 44. Weigh the granules, which pass through sieve No. 20 and are retained on sieve No. 44.
- Add 10% fines (total weight of granules retained on sieve no. 44) to the weighed granules.
- Properly mix the granules with magnesium stearate, talc and remaining quantity of starch.
- Adjust the die cavity as per the desired weight of tablet.
- Compress 2-3 tablets and check the weight.
- Finally compress the granules into the tablets of desired weight.
- Subject the tablets to the various evaluation test mentioned in previous experiments.

Evaluation: To be done as per experiment no 9 (except the disintegration test).

Uniformity of dispersion: The following test is performed for soluble (dispersible) aspirin tablet. Place 1 tablet in 100 ml of water and stir gently until completely dispersed. A smooth dispersion obtained which passes through a sieve screen with a nominal mesh aperture of 710 μm (sieve no 22) without any remains of the dispersed tablet.

Storage: Store in a well closed containers in a cool dry place.

Category: Analgesic, antipyretic, antirheumatic, and antithrombotic.

Dose: As analgesic and antipyretic, 300 to 600 mg four to six times a day.

As antirheumatic, 1 to 2 g four to six times a day.

As antithrombotic 75 mg daily.

Results:

1. **Size:** The average size of tablets was found to be
2. **Shape:** All tablets were spherical/ oval/ oblong in shape.
3. **Weight variation:** Passed/Failed
4. **Hardness:** Average hardness of the tablets was found to be Passed/Failed
5. **% Friabilty:** %Friability was found to be Passed/Failed
6. **Uniformity of dispersion:** Passed/Failed

Precautions

1. Drugs and excipients should be weighed carefully.
2. Weighing paper should be used for weighing of drug and excipients.
3. The overages should be included in the amount of drug and excipients listed in the batch formula to compensate manufacturing loss.
4. Before granulation/or tableting, uniform mixing of drug and excipients should be ensured.
5. Before tableting, punches and tableting station should be cleaned to remove any residue of previous batches.
6. Before tableting, punches should be lubricated with salt of higher fatty acid or with any other lubricants.
7. Working area, punches and punching station should be cleaned before and after granulation/or tableting.

12

To Prepare and Evaluate Chewable Antacid Tablet by a Aqueous Wet Granulation Method

Requirements: Same as previous experiment

Reference: Refer any book given in the list of books at the beginning of this manual.

Formula

S. No.	Ingredients	Quantity per tablet	Quantity taken for 25 tablets
1.	Aluminium hydroxide	400 mg	
2.	Magnesium hydroxide	80 mg	
3.	Sacchrine sodium	20 mg	
4.	Corn starch	10 mg	
5.	Starch paste (5%)	q.s.	
6.	Magnesium stearate	10 mg	
7.	Flavouring agent (Peppermint oil)	q.s.	

Principle

Chewable tablets are chewed and thus mechanically disintegrated in the mouth. The drug is, however, normally not dissolved in the mouth but swallowed and dissolves in the stomach or intestine. Thus, chewable tablets are used primarily to accomplish a quick and complete disintegration of the tablet – and hence obtain a rapid drug effect - or to facilitate the intake of the tablet. Elderly and children in particular have difficulty in swallowing tablets, and so chewable tablets are attractive forms of medication. Important examples are vitamin c tablets, antacid tablets etc.

Chewable tablets are similar in composition to conventional tablets except that a disintegrant is normally not (or low amount) included in the composition. Sweetening agents (Sucrose and mannitol) and colouring agents are commonly used in chewable tablets. The evaluation test of such tablets do not include disintegration test.

In the present experiment aluminium hydroxide and magnesium hydroxide are used for antacid effect. Sucrose is used to provide sweet taste to the chewable preparation. Corn starch is used to disintegrate the tablet and starch paste was used as a binding agent.

Procedure

- Weigh and mix magnesium hydroxide and aluminum hydroxide.
- Dissolve the saccharine sodium in water and combine with starch paste and granulate.
- Dry the granules at 60 °C in an oven and screen through # 16 mesh screen.
- Pass the granules through sieve No. 20 superimposed on sieve No. 44. Weigh the granules, which pass through sieve No. 20 and are retained on sieve No. 44.
- Add 10% fines (total weight of granules retained on sieve no. 44) to the weighed granules.
- Properly mix the granules with flavour, corn starch and magnesium stearate.
- Adjust the die cavity as per the desired weight of tablet.
- Compress 2-3 tablets and check the weight.
- Finally compress the granules into the tablets of desired weight.
- Subject the tablets to the various evaluation test mentioned in previous experiments.

Storage: Store in a well-closed container

Category: Antacid

Dose: 500 mg to 1 g

Evaluation: As per experiment no. 9.

Results: As per experiment no. 11.

Note: Disintegration test is not performed for chewable tablets.

13

To Prepare and Evaluate Aspirin Tablets by Dry Granulation Method

Requirements: Pestle mortar, sieves (# 16), filter paper sheets, hardness tester, friabilator, disintegration apparatus.

Reference: Refer any book given in the list of books at the beginning of this manual.

Formula

S. No.	Ingredients	Quantity per tablet	Quantity taken for 25 tablets
1.	Aspirin	325 mg	
2.	Starch	32.5 mg	
3.	Cab-O-Sil	0.1 mg	

Principle

The method is also known as double compression, slugging, or compression granulation. In the dry methods of granulation the primary powder particles are aggregated/ compacted under high pressure. There are two main processes for such compaction:

Slugging: A large tablet (known as a 'slug') is produced in a heavy-duty tabletting press and the process is known as 'slugging'.

Roller compaction: The powder is squeezed between two rollers to produce a sheet of material and the process is called roller compaction.

In both cases these intermediate products are broken using a suitable milling technique to produce granular material, which is usually sieved to separate the desired size fraction. The unused fine material may be reworked to avoid waste. This dry method may be used for drugs that do not compress well after wet granulation, or those which are sensitive to moisture and heat.

Advantages of dry granulation method

- Less number of processing steps.
- Lower cost.
- Lesser number of excipients.
- No hydrolytic and thermal degradation of sensitive material.

Disadvantages of dry granulation method

- Applicable to limited materials
- Heavy machinery and precise control over pre-compaction.
- Non-uniform mixing of the excipients.
- Difficult in drugs with large doses.
- Difference in particle size and bulk density of the tablet ingredients may leads to non-satisfactory granulation.

Dry granulation technique consists of following steps

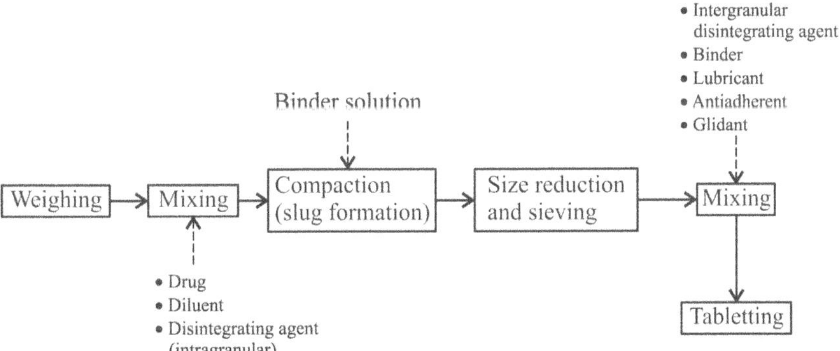

Fig. 13.1 Unit operations in dry granulation tableting method.

Aspirin is the active ingredient in the present formula. Cab-O-Sil (fumed silica) is used as a compressible tablet disintegrant and glidant. Starch is used as filler (diluent) as well as disintegrating agent.

Procedure

- Weigh the desired quantities of the excipients.
- Combine the aspirin, half of the starch and Cab-O-Sil and mix thoroughly.

- Compress the above mixture into slugs using flat face tablet punches.
- Reduce the slugs into granules by passing through sieve no. 16.
- Add remaining quantity of starch to the granules.
- Adjust the die cavity as per the desired weight of tablet.
- Compress the granules into tablets of desired weight.
- Subject the tablets to the various evaluation test as mentioned in experiments no. 9.

Evaluation: As per experiment no. 9.

Storage: Store in a well closed containers in a cool dry place.

Category: Analgesic, antipyretic, antirheumatic, and antithrombotic.

Dose: As analgesic and antipyretic, 300 to 600 mg four to six times a day.

As antirheumatic, 1 to 2 g four to six times a day.

As antithrombotic 75 mg daily.

Results: Same as previous experiment no. 11.

14

To Prepare and Evaluate Acetaminophen Tablets by Direct Compression Method

Requirements: Pestle mortar, filter paper sheets, hardness tester, friabilator, disintegration apparatus.

Reference: Refer any book given in the list of books at the beginning of this manual.

Formula

S. No.	Ingredients	Quantity per tablet	Quantity taken for 25 tablets
1.	Acetaminophen	1325 mg	
2.	Avicel PH 101	1140 mg	
3.	Stearic acid	5 mg	

Principle

A few crystalline substances, such as sodium chloride, potassium chloride, caffeine, citric acid can be compressed directly into tablets. The direct compression method is very simple and has lesser steps than both dry granulation and wet granulation methods. However, only a limited number of drugs have such properties. Further more, the excipients such as diluents, lubricants, disintegrants etc., should also be capable of being directly compressed into tablet.

Advantages of direct compression method

- Less number of processing steps.
- Lower cost.
- No hydrolytic and thermal degradation of sensitive material.

Disadvantages of direct compression method

- Applicable to limited materials.

- Non-uniform mixing of the excipients.

- Difficult in drugs with large doses.

- Difference in particle size and bulk density of the tablet ingredients may leads to non-satisfactory granulation.

- Excipients used are relatively expensive than the excipients used in conventional methods.

Direct compression technique consists of following steps:

Acetaminophen is the active ingredient in the present formula. Avicel PH 101 (Microcrystalline cellulose) is used as a compressible tablet disintegrant and dilluent. Stearic acid is used as glidant.

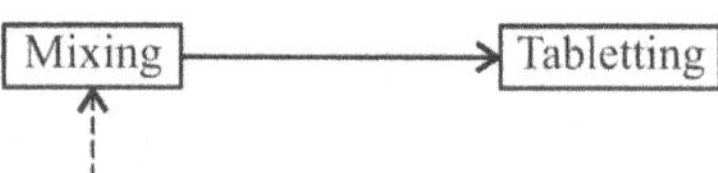

Fig. 14.1 Unit operations in direct compression tableting method.

Procedure

- Weigh desired quantities of all the excipients.

- Combine the acetaminophen and avicel PH 101 and mix thoroughly for 25 min.

- Add fine screened stearic acid to the mixture and mix further for 5 min.

- Adjust the die cavity as per the desired weight of tablet.

- Compress the mixture into tablets of desired weight.

- Subject the tablets to the various evaluation test mentioned in previous experiments.

Evaluation: As per experiment no. 9.

Storage: Store in a well closed containers in a cool dry place.

Category: Analgesic, antipyretic, and antirheumatic.

Dose: As analgesic and antipyretic, 300 to 600 mg three to four times a day.

Results: Same as experiment no. 11.

15

Preparation and Evaluation of Ascorbic Acid Tablets I.P. by Wet Granulation Method using two Different Binders

Requirements: Excipients, pestle mortar, sieves (#10, 20, & 40), hardness tester, friabilator, disintegration apparatus, dissolution apparatus.

Reference: Refer any book given in the list of books at the beginning of this manual.

Formula

S. No.	Ingredients	Quantity per tablet* with ethylcellulose	Quantity per tablet* with methylcellulose
1.	Ascorbic acid	50 mg	50 mg
2.	Lactose	19 mg	19 mg
3.	Starch	15 mg	15 mg
4.	Ethyl cellulose	10 mg	-
5.	Methyl cellulose (MC)	-	10 mg
6.	Talc	5 mg	5 mg
7.	Magnesium stearate	1 mg	1 mg
8.	Alcohol (granulating liquid)	q.s.	-
9.	Water (Granulating liquid)	-	q.s.

*Calculate the quantity of each ingredient for 30 tablets.

Principle

Binders or adhesives are added either in dry or in liquid form to add cohesiveness to powders, thereby providing the necessary bonding to form granules, which under compaction form a cohesive mass or compact referred to as a tablet. The primary criterion when choosing a binder is its compatibility with the other tablet components. Secondarily, it must impart sufficient cohesion to the powders to allow for normal processing (sizing, lubrication, compression, and packaging), yet allow the tablet to disintegrate and the drug to dissolve upon ingestion, releasing the active ingredients for absorption. Examples of various types of binding agents include gum acacia, ethyl cellulose, starch paste, PVP etc.

The tablets are prepared as per experiment no. 10, with two different binders: ethyl cellulose and methyl cellulose. The relative binding efficiency of these agents is evaluated by measuring hardness and disintegration time.

Procedure

Ascorbic acid tablets are prepared in the same way as mentioned in experiment no. 10, but here two different batches are prepared, one batch is prepared using ethyl cellulose as the binder using alcohol as a granulation vehicle while the other batch is prepared using methyl cellulose as the binder and water as a granulating vehicle keeping the remaining ingredients in the formula same.

Evaluation

Evaluation for ascorbic acid tablet is same as mentioned in the experiment no. 9.

Results: Ascorbic acid tablets I.P. were prepared using two different binders viz. ethyl cellulose and methyl cellulose

    (a) Disintegration time: Disintegration time using ethyl cellulose and methyl cellulose was found to be _________ and _________ mins. respectively

    (b) Hardness: Hardness of the tablet prepared using ethyl cellulose and methyl cellulose was found to be _________ and _________ kg/cm^2 respectively.

    (c) Weight variation test: Passed/Failed

    (d) Friability test: % Friability of tablets prepared using ethyl cellulose and methyl cellulose was found to be _________ and _________.

16

To Prepare and Evaluate Mouth Dissolving Tablet of Aspirin by Direct Compression Method

Requirements: Pestle mortar, filter paper sheets, hardness tester, friabilator.

Reference: Refer any book given in the list of books at the beginning of this manual.

Formula

S. No.	Ingredients	Quantity per tablet	Quantity taken for 30 tablets
1.	Aspirin	150 mg	
2.	Sodium starch glycolate	20 mg	
3.	Avicel	88 mg	
4.	Sacchrin	5 mg	
5.	Vanaline	5 mg	
6.	Mannitol	25 mg	
7.	Talc	5 mg	
8.	Mag. Stearate	2 mg	

Principle

Fast dissolving tablets (FDTs) have all the advantages of solid dosage forms, such as good stability, accurate dosing, easy manufacturing, small packaging size, and easy handling by patients. FDTs also have the advantages of liquid formulations, such as easy administration and no risk of suffocation resulting from physical obstruction by a dosage form. The primary patients for FDTs are pediatric, geriatric, and bedridden or developmentally disabled patients; patients with persistent nausea; and patients who have little or no access to water. Application of FDTs can of course be extended to more general patients of daily medication regimens. From the pharmaceutical industry's point of view, FDTs can provide new dosage forms as a life cycle management tool for drugs near the end of their patent life. Because the tablets disintegrate inside the mouth, drugs may be absorbed in the buccal, pharyngeal, and gastric regions resulting into the rapid drug therapy and increased bioavailability. Furthermore, the pre-gastric drug absorption avoids the first-pass metabolism, the drug dose can be reduced if a significant amount of the drug is lost through the hepatic metabolism. FDT are an innovative technology, which disintegrates rapidly, usually in a matter of seconds, without the need for water, providing optimal convenience to the patient. Conventional tablets and capsules pose difficulty for swallowing in patient groups such as elderly, children, and patients mentally retarded, uncooperative, nauseated, or on reduced liquid intake diets. To fulfill the above needs, formulators have devoted considerable efforts for developing FDT. Researchers have formulated FDT for various categories of drugs, which are used for therapy in which rapid peak plasma concentration is required to achieve desired pharmacological response. These include neuroleptics, cardiovascular agents, analgesics, anti-allergic and drugs for erectile dysfunction.

The performance of an FDT depends on the technology used in its manufacture. The disintegrating property of the tablet is attributable to a quick ingress of water into the tablet matrix, which creates porous structure and results in rapid disintegration. Hence, the basic approaches to develop FDT include maximising the porous structure of the tablet matrix, incorporating the appropriate disintegrating agent and using highly water-soluble excipients in the formulation. Techniques, which have been used by various researchers to prepare FDT include Freeze-Drying, Tablet Moulding, Spray Drying, Sublimation, Direct Compression, Cotton Candy Process and Mass-Extrusion. Disintegrating agents are substances routinely included in the tablet formulations to aid in the break up of the compacted mass when it is put into a fluid environment. They promote moisture penetration and dispersion of the tablet matrix. In recent years, several newer agents have been developed known as "Superdisintegrants". These newer substances are more effective at lower concentrations with greater disintegrating efficiency and mechanical strength. On contact with water the superdisintegrants swell, hydrate, change volume or form and produce a disruptive change in the tablet. Effective superdisintegrants provide improved compressibility, compatibility and have no negative impact on the mechanical strength of formulations containing high-dose drugs. Some of the examples of the commonly used superdisintegrants are: crosscamellose sodium, cross-linked polyvinylpyrrolidone, sodium starch glycolate, soy polysaccharide, cross-linked alginic acid, gellan gum, xanthan gum and calcium silicate.

Aspirin is the active ingredient in the present formula. Sodium starch glycolate is used as a superdisintegrant. Avicel PH 101 (Microcrystalline cellulose) is used as a dilluent. Saccharin, vanalline and mannitol are used to enhance the taste. Talc and magnesium stearate are used as glidant.

Procedure

As per experiment no. 14.

Evaluation: As per experiment no. 9.

Except the following test is applicable only to dispersible tablets.

Method (Uniformity of Dispersion)

- Place 1 tablets in 100 ml of water and stir gently until completely dispersed.

- A smooth dispersion is obtained which passes through a sieve screen with a normal mesh aperture of 710 um (sieve no. 22) without any remains of the dispersed tablet.

Storage: Store in a well closed containers in a cool dry place.

Category: Analgesic, antipyretic, antirheumatic, and antithrombotic.

Dose: As analgesic and antipyretic, 300 to 600 mg three to four times a day.

Results: As per experiment no. 11.

PHARMA TRIVIA: SELF EVALUATION TEST

1. Enlist ingredient of an effervescent tablets.
2. Name a few directly compressible tablet diluents.
3. What is the concentration range of colloidal silica used as glidant?
4. Which part in a tablet compression machine, guides the movement of punches?
5. Give the formula for Hausner ratio?
6. What is the range of angle of repose for good flow?
7. Name any four tablet defects.
8. How can capping of tablet be eliminated?
9. Punch faces in the tableting machine are coated with which element for producing smooth non adherent face?
10. What is Carr's compressibility index?
11. Why aspirin tablets are made by non-aqueous granulation method?
12. Name any three enteric coating substances.
13. What are the differences in composition of normal tablet and chewable tablets?
14. What is the difference in shape between upper and lower punches?
15. Name official test for evaluation of tablets under USP and IP?
16. What are super-disintegrants? Give two examples.
17. Why lactose is not used as a diluent in tablets containing paracetamol?
18. Name any two devices for evaluation of hardness of tablets.
19. What is the concentration range of disintegrating agent used in tablet manufacturing?
20. Write down any two major differences between single station and multi station tablet compression machines?

4

Coating of Granules

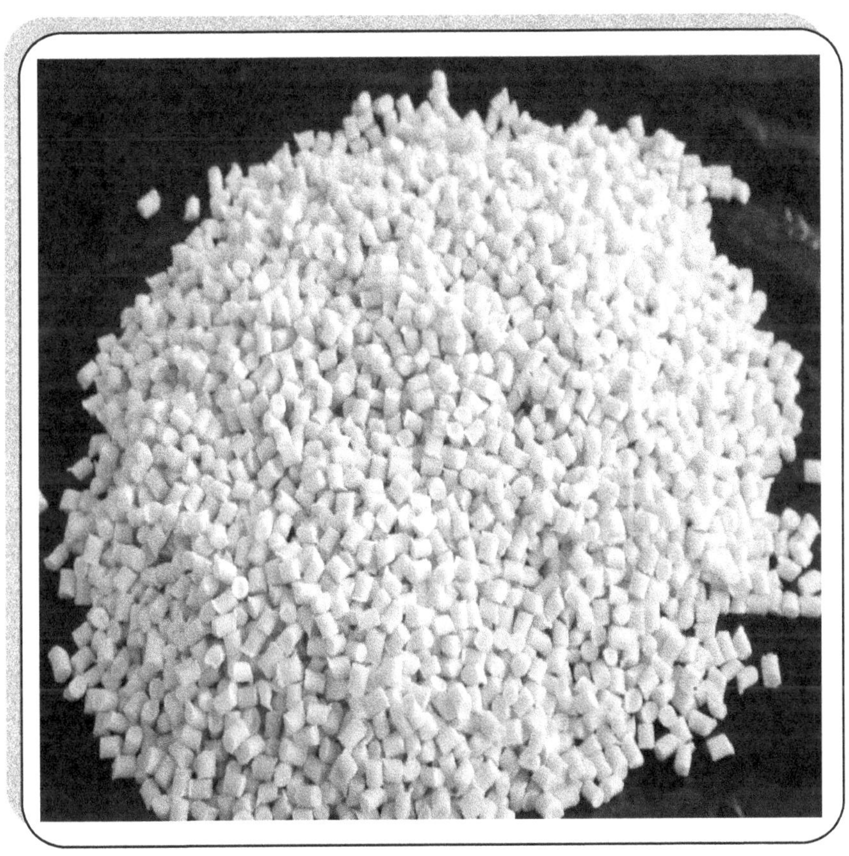

Tablet coating is a process in which an edible material is applied to the surface of a solid pharmaceutical dosage form. This edible material may be sugar (Sugar coating) or polymers (Film coating). Traditionally sugar coating was a common solution for coating tablets, but due to some disadvantages, modern tablet coatings are typically film coatings, which can be applicable to wide range of dosage forms (such as tablets, capsules, pellets, granules and drug particles). There are three major components of coating process:

1. Core material (Drug)
2. Coating material (Film former)
3. Coating equipments

Applications

1. To mask the taste, odor or color of the drug.
2. To provide the physical and chemical protection for the drug.
3. To control the release of the drug from tablet.
4. To protect the drug from gastric environment of stomach with an acid resistant coating.
5. To improve the pharmaceutical elegance by use of special colorus and contrast printing.
6. To incorporate another drug or adjuncts in coating to avoid the chemical incompatibilities.
7. To protect the drug from environmental conditions (Oxygen, moisture and light).

PHARMACEUTICAL COATING PROCESSES

Tablet coating is the application of a coating composition to a moving bed of tablets with the concurrent use of heated air to facilitate the evaporation of solvent.

The major coating techniques are:

1. Sugar coating
2. Film coating
3. Micro encapsulation
4. Compression coating (solvent organic/water) is absent
5. Dip coating
6. Vacuum coating

Core materials: It may be

1. Drug/active constituent
2. Flavoring agent
3. Coloring agent
4. Stabilizers
5. Taste masking agents
6. Incompatible material

Coating materials

(i) Sugar and sugar substitute
    (a) Ex:glucose, Lactose, mannitol, sorbitol etc
(ii) Water soluble polymers as film former
    (b) Ex: Polyethylene Glycol(PEG), Polyvinyl pyrrolidone (PVP), Sodium carboxymethyl cellulose(NaCMC) etc.
(iii) Polymers of modified dissolution and disintegration properties.
    (c) Ex: Cellulose Acetate Phthalate (CAP), Zien, Shellac, Hydroxypropylmethyl cellulose phthalate (HPMCP) etc.

Coating Equipments

Most coating processes use three major types of coating equipments

1. Standard coating pan
2. Perforated coating pan
3. Fluidized bed coating pan (Air Suspension method)

Coating Process Variables

1. Size and shape of core material
2. Quantity of core material
3. Size of coating pan
4. Speed of rotation of coating pan
5. Nature and concentration of coating material.
6. Viscosity of coating solution
7. Temperature during coating process
8. Rate of spray of coating solution

17

To Prepare and Evaluate the Control Release Granules of Ascorbic Acid by Pan Coating Method

Requirements: Ascorbic acid, conventional coating pan, beaker, stirrer, measuring cylinder, glass rod etc.

Reference: Refer any book given in the list of books at the beginning of this manual.

Formula: Formula for coating solution:

Material Name	Weight (% w/v)	Use
HPMC	6	Film-forming polymer
PEG 400	2	Plasticizer
PEG 6000	2	Alloying
Dye	0.24	Colorant
Titanium dioxide	2	Opaquant
Water q.s.	q.s.	Vehicle

Principle

Coating pans made from stainless steels or copper with diameter from 8 to 60 inches are used. The pan is mounted on the drive from a variable speed motor. The pan must also be provided with hot and cold air supply duct and an exhaust duct for removal of vapor and dust generated during the coating operation.

The core materials greater than 600 μ in size and spherical in shape are generally considered essential for effective coating and process has been extensively employed for the preparation of controlled release beads. Core material are carried upwards by the rotation of pan until their centrifugal and frictional forces are overcome by gravity causing individual cores to roll and fall away form surface of the bed (Cascading movements). A system of properly designed baffles may be fitted to the inside of the pan to improve the uniformity of tumbling or cascading action in the pan. Coating solutions are applied to the tablets by ladling or spraying the coating material onto the rotating tablet bed.

Advantages

(a) The process may be employed to apply a wide variety of nonenteric and enteric film formers together with other additives such as plasticizer and colorants in organic solvent or aqueous based systems.

(b) The great flexibility in the formulation of the coating.

(c) Core material may also contain a wide range of additives that serve to modify further the release properties of the final dosage form.

Disadvantages

(a) Technical difficulties in obtaining satisfactory coating and because large number of variables some of which are not easily controlled, that affect coating quality.

(b) Lack of consistency and reproducibility.

(c) Production times of a week or more.

Method of preparation

- Place the weighed amount of ascorbic acid granules (particle size $\geq$ 500 μ) in the conventional coating pan. (Please refer Experiment no 10 for Ascorbic acid granules).

- Optimize the speed of rotation of coating pan to ensure the free movement of granules (cascading movement).

- Fill the spray gun with coating solution.

- Pass the hot air to coating pan at the desirable temperature and rate.

- Spray the coating solution on granule bed and dry the granules.

- Weigh the final coated granules and calculate the coating efficiency.

Ascorbic granules prepared by Wet/Dry granulation technique can be used for this purpose (experiment no. 12 and 13).

Evaluation

1. Organoleptic Properties

    Color

    Odor

    Taste

    Sticking

    Uniformity of colour

2. Size and shape: By microscopic method/ Sieving method

3. Coating efficiency:

    Net increase in coated tablet weight = Final weight of coated tablets
    − Initial weight of uncoated tablets

$$\text{Coating efficiency}(E) = \frac{\text{Net increase in coated tablet weight}}{\text{weight of the coating material}} \times 100$$

Results:

1. Organoleptic properties: Granules were found to be of spherical and uniform in color.
2. Size: Average size of granules was found to be ________ mm
3. Coating efficiency: It was found to be ________ %

Precautions

1. Solid core particles greater than 500 µ are generally considered necessary for satisfactory coating.
2. The core should be spherical in shape so as to roll well in coating pan, for this, spherical substrate (nonpareil / sugar pellets) is used.
3. They should be adequately hard and of low friability so as to withstand attrition during the process.

PHARMA TRIVIA: SELF EVALUATION TEST

1. Write the name of two polymers used in film coating
2. What do you mean by seal coat?
3. Write the two examples of enteric coated polymers.
4. Write the name of different methods involved in coating technology.
5. Write the disintegration time of enteric coated and uncoated tablets.
6. Give the suitable example of acrylate polymer.
7. What are the problems associated with film coating and sugar coating.
8. What do you understand by atomization?
9. What are the materials required for sugar coating?
10. Give the name of materials required to reduce sticking or picking of granules.
11. What are the factors affecting coating process?
12. Define mottling and orange peel.
13. Enumerate various steps involved in sugar coating.
14. Name any two coating pans.
15. Write down the formula for % coating efficiency.

5

Capsules

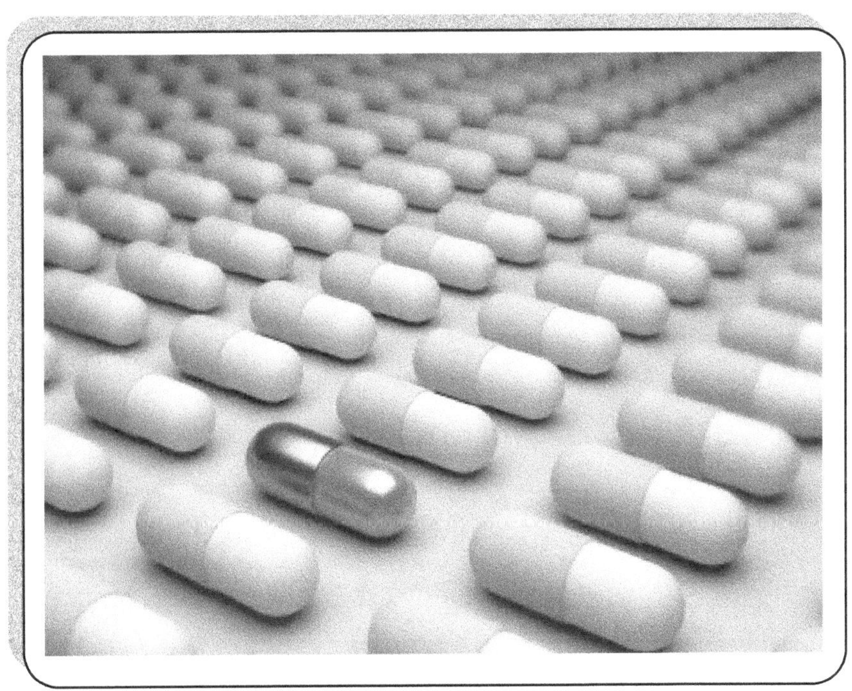

Capsules are solid dosage forms in which the drug is enclosed within either a hard or soft soluble container or "shell". Capsules are solid preparations with hard or soft shells of various shapes and capacities, usually containing a single dose of active substance(s). They are intended for oral administration. The shells are usually formed from gelatin; however, they may also be made from starch, cellulose or other suitable substances.

Types of Capsule Shell

1. Hard gelatin capsules
2. Soft gelatin capsules
3. Modified-release capsules (including delayed-release capsules (gastro-resistant/enteric capsules) and sustained-release capsules (extended-/prolonged-release capsules).

Table 5.1 Difference between hard and soft gelatin capsule

Hard gelatin capsule (HGC)	Soft gelatin capsule (SGC)
1. Hard in the nature.	Soft in the nature.
2. Consist two parts – body and cap.	It is a single entity.
3. Manufactured in two stages – shells are prepared first and then filling is done afterwards.	Manufactured in one stage i.e., preparation of shell and filling is done simultaneously.
4. Contains less amount of plasticizer so less elastic in nature.	Contains high amount of plasticizer so more elastic in nature.
5. Generally used for filling solid materials.	Used for filling solid, liquid and semisolid preparations.
6. Available in only one shape	Available in different shapes
7. Time consuming	Fast process
8. Non Tamper proof	Tamper proof

Composition of Capsule Shell

The shell of hard gelatin capsules basically consists of gelatin, plasticizers, preservatives and water (**primary components**). Modern day shells may, in addition, consist of colours, opacifying agents, flavours, sugars, acids, enteric materials etc (**secondary components**). The gelatin is marketed in a large number of varieties and a specific quality of gelatin having specified gel strength, viscosity, iron content etc., should be selected for capsules. Gelatin is major component of the capsule which is available in nature and widely used due to its advantages like:

1. Non toxic and widely used in foodstuffs.
2. World-wide acceptable.
3. Easy soluble in biological fluid at body temperature.
4. Good film forming material.
5. As a solution in water or glycerol water blend, it undergoes a irreversible phase change from sol. to gel.

Source of gelatin: gelatin is obtained from the following sources:

1. Animal bones (bone gelatin) produce a tough firm film but tends to hazy and brittle.
2. Animal skin (skin gelatin) obtained from frozen calf and pork skin. It gives plasticity and clarity to shell and thereby reducing haze or cloudiness in the finished capsules.

It is prepared by hydrolysis of collagen which is main protein constituents of connective tissue. Physical and chemical properties of gelatin are the function of:

1. Parent collagen
2. Method of extraction
3. pH value
4. Thermal degradation
5. Electrolyte content.

Types of Gelatin

Type A: Produced by acid precursor and isoelectric point in the region of pH 9.

Type B: Produced by alkali treated precursor and isoelectric point in region of pH 4.7.

Following properties of gelatin must be considered for manufacturing of capsule shell.

1. Bloom strength.
2. Viscosity
3. Iron content

Bloom Strength: It is a measure of cohesive strength of crosslinking that occurs between gelatin molecules and is proportional to the molecular weight of gelatin.

The ideal range of the bloom strength is 150-250 g. It is directly proportional to physical stability (high bloom strength, physically more stable capsule shell and cost is also high and shell is used when necessary to improve the physical stability of product.

e.g: large capsule (50 minim)

Viscosity: The viscosity of the gelatin is determined on a 6.66% concentration of gelatin in water at 60^0C and is a measure of molecular chain length. The ideal range of the viscosity for gelatin is 25 to 45 mp. (38 ± 2 mp). Thickness of shell depends on viscosity.

Iron: Present in raw gelatin and concentration usually depends on the water used for its manufacturing.

Plasticizer: It gives the particular elasticity or flexibility to capsule shell. Some of the commonly used plasticizers are glycerin, sorbitol, acacia, sucrose and polyethylene glycol (PEG). The ratio of dry gelatin to dry plasticizer determines the hardness of gelatin shell. In the hard gelatin the ratio of dry gelatin to dry plasticizer is 1:0.4; while in the soft gelatin capsule the ratio is 1:0.8.

Preservatives: Preservative is added to capsule as in process aid in order to prevent microbiological contamination. During manufacturing moisture level should be such that it will not support bacterial growth. The commonly used preservatives are: methyl paraben and propyl paraben.

Hard gelatin capsule shell is prepared by mold pin dipping method, which is automatic process and contains various steps like: dipping-spinning-drying-stripping-trimming-joining the capsule. The capsule shells should be stored under controlled conditions of temperature and humidity. The normal moisture content of shell is 10 to 15%. Under conditions of low humidity they may soften and grow tacky.

Advantages

1. The shells are physiologically inert, easily and quickly digested in the gastro intestinal tract.
2. They are slippery when moist and hence easy to swallow with a draught of water.
3. They are elegant and attractive in appearance.
4. They obscure the taste and odor of unpleasant drugs.
5. The shells can be opacified (with titanium dioxide) or colored, to give protection from light.

6. If properly stored the shell contain 12-15% of moisture which gives flexibility and consequently considerable resistance to mechanical stress.

7. Less adjuncts are necessary than for tablets.

8. Provides substantial protection against air and moisture.

Limitations

1. Capsules are generally not used for administration of extremely soluble material for example - ammonium chloride (NH_4Cl), potassium chloride (KCl) and potassium bromide (KBr). Since sudden release of such compounds in stomach could result in irritation in stomach.

2. Not used for highly efflorescent or deliquescent materials because such material may cause the capsule to soften whereas deliquescent powder may dry the capsule shell to excessive brittleness.

3. Shells become brittle, when the moisture content of the shell is decreased.

4. Some drugs can interact with amino groups of gelatin protein.

5. Storage under severe conditions, cause gelatin to crosslink and thereby reducing solubility of the capsule shell.

6. Gelatin capsule shells are mainly of bovine origin, which creates a theoretical risk of transmitting bovine spongiform encephalopathy (BSE) via capsules.

7. Religious or vegetarian dietary restrictions.

8. Sometimes shell may adhere to esophagus.

Pharmaceutical Applications

1. As an oral dosage form of proprietary product for human and veterinary use.

2. As suppository dosage form for rectal or for vaginal use.

3. As special package in tube form for human and veterinary single dose application of topical, ophthalmic and otic preparation and rectal ointments.

4. In cosmetic industry these capsule may be used as special package for breath fresheners, perfumes, bath oil and various skin creams.

18

To Evaluate Empty Hard Gelatin Capsules

Requirements: Empty gelatin capsule (large size if possible), petri plate, vernier calipers, balance, forceps, oven, disintegration apparatus.

Reference: Refer any book given in the list of books at the beginning of this manual.

Principle

The manufacturing and filling processes for capsules should meet the requirements of good manufacturing practices (GMP). Very broad guidelines are available which has to be followed during production of capsules.

Quality control tests are divided into:

Physical Test includes capsule size, integrity of the seals, the moisture content of shell as well as the mixture, disintegration and weight variation.

Chemical Test includes dissolution test, Assay, Stability, Content uniformity.

Procedure

Take 20 capsules of same size and color. Evaluate the capsules for following parameters:

1. **The surface characteristics**
    (a) Type of capsules: Hard/Soft
    (b) Color: Transparent, Red and Black, Blue, Blue/Black

(c) Elegance: Elegant/Nonelegant

(d) Mottling: Present/Absent

(e) Presence of pin holes: Present/Absent

(f) Orange peeling or gritty particles: Present/Absent

(g) Tackiness: Tacky/Nontacky

(h) Body to cap contact: Tight/Loose/Ideal

(i) Edges of body and cap: Rough/Smooth

2. **Dimensional variation:** Measure the length of body and cap of each capsule with the help of vernier calipers.

3. **Weight variation:** Take 20 capsules and weigh it. Find out the average weight. Calculate ±10% of average weight*. Now weigh 20 capsules individually.

> *** Official limit** = ±10%. or ± 7.5% of average weight

1. If average weight of capsule is less than 300 mg ($\leq$ 300 mg), apply ±10% variation of average weight
2. If the average weight of capsule is more than 300 mg ($\geq$ 300 mg) apply ± 7.5% variation of average weight.

Observations and Calculation

Weight of 20 capsules = A gms

Average weight of capsule = A/20 = B gms

If the average weight (B) is $\leq$ 300 mg, apply ±10% variation of average weight

For ± 10% of average weight,

$$B \times 10/100 = C$$

So, $\quad B + C = D$ gm and

$\quad B - C = E$ gm

Range of Weight variation – D gm to E gm

Table 18.1 Weight variation test

S. No.	Weight of Capsule (gm)	% weight variation	Result (Passed/Failed)
1.			
2.			
3.			
4.			
5.			

Table 18.1 *Contd...*

6.			
7.			
8.			
9.			
10.			
11.			
12.			
13.			
14.			
15.			
16.			
17.			
18.			
19.			
20.			

The range for weight variation is D gm to E gm. If more than 2 capsules are out of the range, the test is failed.

Moisture content:

- Weigh an empty Petri-plate (with its cover) = ... gm
- Put 20 capsules in it and weigh = ... gm
- Calculate the weight of 20 capsules.
- Keep Petri plate in an oven at 60 °C and weigh after 2 minutes.
- Repeat this process till two consecutive readings are same.
- This shows complete drying of capsules.
- Calculate percentage moisture content by using following formula

% Moisture content = Initial weight of capsules – Final weight of capsules/Initial weight of capsules × 100

Observations and Calculation

1. At room temperature

Weight of empty petri plate = A gm

Weight of 20 capsules + Petri plate = B gm

So, weight of 20 capsules = B – A = C gm (Initial reading at room temperature)

2. At 60 °C

Weight of 20 capsules at 60 °C after 2 minutes = D gm

Weight of 20 capsules at 60 °C after 4 minutes = E gm

Weight of 20 capsules at 60 °C after 6 minutes = F gms

Weight of 20 capsules at 60 °C after 8 minutes = G gms (G & F are same in this case)

% Moisture content = C – G/C × 100 = …… %

Official limit = 10 to 15 %

Disintegration test: Perform the test on 6 capsules of each batch at 37 °C. Attach a steel wire helix (sinker) to the capsule in order to prevent floating of capsules (For detail procedure refer Experiment No. 5). Note time for each capsule at which it breaks into pieces and no material is left on the screen. Calculate average Disintegration time.

Official limit = Up to 30 minutes

Results:

1. **Visual Inspection:** The visual inspection has been performed.
2. **Dimensional variation:** Average length of the body and cap of capsules was   found to be ________ mm and ________ mm.
3. **Weight variation:** Passed/Failed.
4. **Moisture content:** The moisture content of capsules was found to be ________ %.
5. **Disintegration time:** The average disintegration time of capsules was found to be ________ min.

Precautions

1. Do not touch capsules with bare hand. Always use forceps or wear gloves.
2. For moisture content determination in capsule shell, lid of petri dishes should be closed while taking out the capsule shell from hot air oven.
3. For moisture content determination temperature should not exceed 50 °C.

19

To Determine the Size and Filling Capacity (Displacement Value) of Hard Gelatin Capsule in Relation to the Given Diluents

Requirements: 20 capsules of same size and color;

Drug: (aspirin/paracetamol/amoxycillin/ferrous sulphate/aluminium hydroxide, magnesium sulphate/ferrous sulphate;

Diluents: (lactose/starch/calcium phosphate/calcium dihydrogen phosphate/sorbitol/mannitol/MCC) etc.

Reference: Refer any book given in the list of books at the beginning of this manual.

Principle

The average capsule volume and capsule filled weight capacity for powder dose densities varies with capsule size. They are available in nine sizes, identified by numbers ranging from 000 (largest) to 5 (smallest). The standard industrial sizes used today for human medicines are from 0-4. Their capacities vary with the density of the contents and the pressure applied during filling. To estimate the size of the capsules in terms of the volume of the capsule shell is determined by dividing the filled weight for a powder by its tapped bulk density. A filled weight capacity for the typical powder for different capsule size is given in the Table 19.1:

Table 19.1 Capacities of different capsule shell

Capsule sizes	Capsule volume (cc or ml)	Capsule weight capacity in mg			
		Powder dose density			
		0.6 g/cc	0.8 g/cc	1.0 g/cc	1.2 g/cc
000	1.37	822	1096	1370	1644
00	0.95	570	760	950	1140
0 el	0.78	468	624	780	36
0	0.68	408	544	680	816
1	0.50	300	400	500	600
2	0.37	222	296	370	444
3	0.30	180	240	300	360
4	0.21	126	168	210	252
5	0.13	78	104	130	156

As the volume occupied by the drug and excipients varies as per their density, it is important to calculate the weight of the excipients for each drug. Displacement method is used to calculate the amount of excipients required to fill in the capsule for a given dose of the drug. A "displacement value" is calculated as per the capacity of capsule shell to accommodate the filling material. The displacement value is further used to calculate the weight of the excipients to be filled. It is calculated by the following formula:

$$\text{Displacement value (D)} = \frac{\text{Amount of diluent in one capsule}}{\text{Amount of drug in one capsule}}$$

Procedure

(i)   Calculation of displacement value:

- Take 20 capsules and weigh it.
- Remove cap from each capsule, fill body with given diluent and weigh it.
- Remove the diluents and again fill the capsules with the given drug and weigh.

Observations

Weight of 20 empty capsules	=	X gm
Weight of 20 capsules with diluent	=	Y gm
Weight of 20 capsules with drug	=	Z gm

Calculations

$$\text{Amount of diluent in 1 capsule} = \frac{Y-X}{20} = A$$

$$\text{Amount of drug in 1 capsule} = \frac{Z-X}{20} = B$$

$$\text{Displacement value (D)} = \frac{\text{Amount of diluent in one capsule } (A)}{\text{Amount of drug in one capsule } (B)}$$

Calculation of Size of Capsule

Procedure

- Take 20 gm of drug and put into a dry and clean measuring cylinder.
- Tap the cylinder until the volume become constant and note down the volume (tapped volume).
- Calculate the tap density by using following formula:

Tapped density (⌐) = Weight of the drug/ Tapped volume (Size of capsule)

Size of capsule (Tapped volume) = Weight of drug in one capsule (B gm)/Tapped density (⌐)

Results:

(i)   Displacement value of given capsule was found to be _________

(ii) The size (volume) of the capsule shell was found to be _________ (refer capsule volume table given in theory part)

Precautions

1. Do not touch capsules with bare hand. Always use forceps or wear gloves.
2. Disc or sinker should be used while performing disintegration test.
3. Before filling of the capsules, uniform mixing of drug and excipients should be ensured.
4. For manual filling of capsule shells, filling should be done with uniform tapping.

5. Working area should be cleaned before and after filling of capsules.

6. After filling, capsule shell should be clean with muslin cloth or cotton ball.

Application

Designing of formula for capsule formulation.

20

To Study the Optimization of Formula for Capsule Dosage form using Different Drugs and Excipients for a given Dose (25/50/75/100 mg) and their Evaluation

Requirements: 20 capsules of same size and color, drug (aspirin/magnesium sulphate/paracetamol etc.), measuring cylinder, balance, diluents (starch/lactose etc.), glidient (talc/magnesium stearate/ stearic acid etc.).

Reference: Refer any book given in the list of books at the beginning of this manual.

Principle

Hard gelatin capsules can be filled with a large variety of materials of different physicochemical properties. All materials for filling into capsules have to meet the following basic requirements:

- Must not react with gelatin.
- Must not contain a high level of 'free' moisture.
- Volume of the unit dose must not exceed the sizes of capsule available.
- Must be capable of being filled uniformly to give a stable product.
- Must release their active contents in a form that is available for absorption by the patient.

- Must comply with the requirements of the Pharmacopoeias and regulatory authorities, e.g., dissolution tests.

The majority of products for filling into capsules are formulated as powders. These are typically mixtures of the active ingredient together with a combination of different types of excipients like:

Diluents, which give plug-forming properties

Lubricants, which reduce powder to metal adhesion

Glidants, which improve powder flow

Wetting agents, which improve water penetration

Disintegrants, which produce disruption of the powder mass

Stabilizers, which improve product stability

The selection of the excipients depends upon several factors such as:

- The properties of the active drug, its dose, solubility, particle size and shape.
- The size of capsule to be used.
- The filling machines to be used.

The size of the capsules defines the free space inside the capsule that is available to the formulator. The easier active compounds to formulate are low-dose potent ones, which in the final formulation occupy only a small percentage of the total volume - <20% and so the properties of the mixture will be governed by the excipients chosen, whereas those compounds with a high unit dose, e.g., 500 mg of an antibiotic, leave little free space within the capsule and excipients must be chosen that exert their effect at low concentrations, <5%, and the properties of the mixture will be governed by that of the active ingredient. There are three main factors in powder formulation:

- Good flow, (using free-flowing diluent and glidant).
- No adhesion (using lubricant).
- Cohesion (plug-forming diluent).
- Uniform size and size distribution.
- Should be free from electrostatic charges.

The factor that contributes most to the uniform filling of capsules is good powder flow. This is because the powder bed, from which the dose is measured, needs to be homogeneous and packed reproducibly in order to achieve uniform fill weights.

The filling of the capsules is basically divided into two type: batch scale or small scale filling and industrial or the large scale filling. The major difference between the available methods is the way in which the dose of material is measured into the capsule body. The industrial scale filling can be divided into the two groups:

Dependent dosing systems: Use the capsule body directly to measure the powder. Uniformity of fill weight can only be achieved if the capsule is filled completely.

Example: Auger

Independent dosing systems: The powder is measured independently of the body in a special measuring device. Weight uniformity is not dependent on filling the body completely. With this system the capsule can be part filled.

Example: Dossator, tamping figure and dosing disc.

Procedure

(i) **Calculation of the filling capacity:** As per experiment no 19.

(ii) **Calculation of amount of diluents for the given dose:**
Amount of diluent in one capsule (D) =
(Amount of drug in one capsule – dose) × filling capacity

(iii) **Calculation of amount of glidant for the given dose:**
Amount of glidant (1%) in one capsule (G) =
(Amount of diluent in one capsule (D) + dose) ×1/100

Table 20.1 Optimization of the formula

S. No.	Excipients	Quantity calculated for one capsule	Quantity calculated for 20 capsules
	Drug	Dose of the drug	
	Diluent	......mg	
	Glidant	.......mg	

(iv) **Formulation of the capsule:**

- Weigh the drug and excipients for the 20 capsules (calculate for 1 or 2 extra capsules).
- Mix properly and fill into the capsules.
- Clean the capsule surface with muslin cloth.
- Evaluate the capsules for weight variation and disintegration.

Results:

- Weight of diluent in one capsule = _________ mg
- Weight of glidant in one capsule = _________ mg
- Weight variation test = Passed/failed
- Disintegration time _________ min

Precautions

Same as previous experiment.

Application: Same as previous experiment.

21

To Prepare and Evaluate the antacid Capsules of Magnesium Oxide and Sodium Bicarbonate (1:1)

Requirements: 20 capsules of same size, antacid mixture, diluents.

Reference: Refer any book given in the list of books at the beginning of this manual.

Principle

In the present experiment, mixture of magnesium oxide and sodium carbonate is used as an antacid. Magnesium oxide (MgO), or magnesia, is a white hygroscopic solid mineral and is used for relief of heartburn, sore stomach, magnesium supplement and as a short-term laxative. It is also used to improve symptoms of indigestion. Sodium bicarbonate is used as an antacid to treat heartburn, indigestion, and stomach upset. Sodium bicarbonate is a very quick-acting antacid. It should be used only for temporary relief. In-process controls during hard capsule production include the moisture content of the mixture and/or granulate (as well as of the shells), the size of granules, the flow of the final mixture and the uniformity of mass, capsule size, integrity of the seals and disintegration or dissolution rate (e.g., for modified-release capsules) of the finished dosage form.

Procedure

- Prepare the antacid mixture by taking Magnesium oxide and Sodium bicarbonate in ratio 1:1.
- Mix thoroughly and keep it aside.

- Now weigh 20 empty gelatin capsules.
- Fill with diluent (lactose) and weigh again.
- Remove the diluent and again fill the capsules with the prepared antacid mixture and weigh.
- Calculate the filling capacity, amount of diluents, amount of lubricant in one capsule, and optimize the formula (as given in previous experiment for 1 capsule).
- Then calculate the quantity of each excipients for 20 capsule.
- Weigh and properly mix all the excipients and fill into capsule shells.
- Perform weight variation test on 20 capsules.

Calculation

Same as experiment no. 19.

Results:

1. Displacement value of given capsule was found to be _______.
2. Antacid capsules prepared and evaluated for weight variation test. Capsules passed/failed the weight variation test.

Precautions

Same as previous experiment.

Application: Same as previous experiment.

PHARMA TRIVIA: SELF EVALUATION TEST

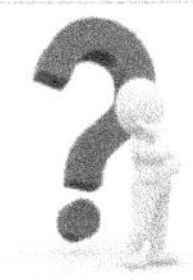

1. What makes the shell of soft gelatin capsules, elastic or plastic in nature?
2. What is the function of sulphur dioxide used in gelatin preparation?
3. What is displacement value? Give formula.
4. What are the different components of capsule shell?
5. Which capsule filling machine is based on auger fill principle?
6. What is bloom strength?
7. What are the values of bloom strength for hard gelatin and soft gelatin capsule?
8. Name one opacifying agent used in capsule shells.
9. What are pearls?
10. What is the difference between pharmagel A and pharmagel B?
11. What are the advantages and disadvantages of capsules over tablets?
12. What are the various evaluation parameters for capsules?
13. Which kinds of materials are dispensed into soft gelatin capsules?
14. Define base absorption.
15. What are the important characteristics of drug/excipients which affect their filling capacity?

6

Microencapsulation

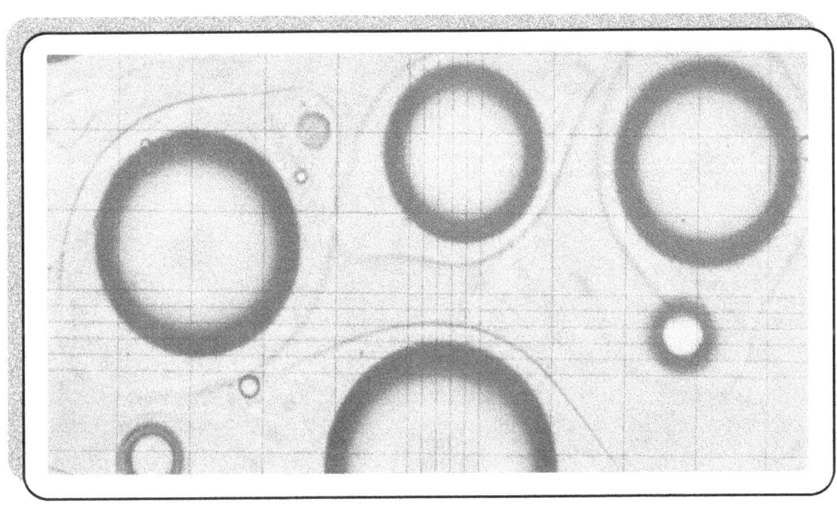

Microencapsulation is the process of applying relatively thin coatings to small particles of solids or droplets of liquids and dispersion to produce microcapsule (1-5000 μ). Microcapsules are tiny particles that contain an active agent or core material surrounded by a shell or coating, and are now increasingly being used in food ingredients preparation. Microencapsulation technology can be used to deliver a host of ingredients - flavours, oils, peptides, amino acids, enzymes, acidulants, colours and sweeteners - in a range of food formulations, from functional foods to ice cream.

The technology can also decrease costs for food makers, particularly those using sensitive ingredients like probiotics, and by reducing the need for preservatives.

Microencapsulation has been widely used for the encapsualtion of many products such as:

- Molecules (antibiotic, antigen, dye, enzyme)
- Virus
- Bacteria (Lactobacillus, Pseudomonas)
- Cells (Langherans islets, hepatocytes ...)

Advantages

1. Microencapsulation provides a means for converting liquids to solids of altering colloidal and surface properties.
2. To improve the stability by providing environmental protection against light, moisture and oxygen.
3. Because of smallness of particles, drug can be widely distributed throughout GI tract thereby potentially improving drug absorption (Bioavailability).
4. It provides sustained released or prolonged action medications.
5. To mask unpleasanr taste, odor and color.
6. It is also used in formulation of single layer tablet containing incompatible ingredients.
7. Pharmaceutical related areas such as hygiene, diagnostic aids and medical equipment design also are amenable to micro-encapsulation application.

Drawbacks

1. The release characteristic of coated product is not always reproducible.
2. The coating may often be discontinuous.
3. No single technique can be adapted to all core materials.
4. In the case of very sensitive pharmaceuticals the shelf life would be inadequate.
5. Higher cost may be stumbling block in its application.

Fundamental Consideration

The technique involves basic understanding of the general properties of microcapsule such as.

1. Nature of the core and coating materials.
2. The stability and release characteristics of the coated materials.
3. Microencapsulation methods.

Types of Microencapsulation Process

There are three microencapsulation processes. They are:

I.   Chemical process

1. Interfacial polymerization
2. In-situ polymerization
3. Orifice method - (for solid and liquids).

II.   Physico-chemical processes

1. Phase separation coacervation
2. Complex coacervation
3. Complex emulsion
4. Meltable dispersion
5. Powder bed.

III. Mechanical process

1. Air suspension or fluidized bed coating (for solids)
2. Pan coating (for solids)
3. Spray drying (for solids)
4. Spray congealing (for liquids)
5. Electrostatic bonding.

Table 6.1 Different microencapsulation process and their applicabilities

Microencapsulation	Application core material	Approximate particlesize (μ m)
➢ Air suspension	Solids	35-5000*
➢ Coacervation-phase separation.	Solids and liquids	2-5000*
	Solids and liquids	1-5000*
➢ Multiorifice centrifugal	Solids	600-5000*
➢ Pan coating	Solids and liquids	5-5000*
➢ Solvent evaporation	Solids and liquids	6000*
➢ Spray drying and congealing		

*5000-µm size is not a particle limitation. The methods are also applicable for macrocoating i.e., particle size greater than 5000 µ.

22

To Prepare and Evaluate Sustained Release Granules of Ascorbic Acid (By Phase-Separation Coacervation Technique - Microencapsulation)

Requirements: Glass beaker, glass rod, water bath, hot plate/heater, icebath, dissolution apparatus (I.P. 1).

References: Refer any book given in the list of books at the beginning of this manual.

Formula

S. No.	Ingredients	Quantity given	Quantity taken
1.	Ascorbic acid	4 gm	
2.	Ethyl cellulose	2 gm	
3.	Cyclohexane	100 ml	

Principle

Microencapsulation is a technology devoted to entrapping solids, liquids, or gases inside one or more polymeric coatings. There are number of encapsulation methods, which include interfacial polymerization, complex coacervation, coacervation, thermal denaturation, salting-out, solvent evaporation, hot melt, solvent removal, spray-drying and spray congealing. In present experiment coacervation phase separation is used to prepare the ascorbic acid microcapsules.

Microencapsulation by coacervation phase separation consists of 3 steps:

1. **Formation of 3 immiscible chemical phases**: liquid manufacturing vehicle phase, core material phase & coating material phase

2. **Deposition of the coating material around the core:** Deposition of liquid polymer coating around core by polymer adsorbed at the interface formed between core material and vehicle phase

3. **Rigidization of coating:** Coating material is immiscible in vehicle phase and it gets rigidized over the core material. This could be achieved by thermal, cross-linking, or dissolvation techniques.

In the present experiment phase separation coacervation micro-encapsulation was carried out by using temperature variation. Ascorbic acid is the core material and ethyl cellulose is the coating polymer. Ethyl cellulose dissolves in cyclohexane at higher temperature but precipitate out at lower temperature. A solution of ethyl cellulose in cyclohexane is deposited over ascorbic acid core at lower temperature and finally the rigidization is carried out by cooling the mixture to room temperature.

Procedure

- Disperse ethyl cellulose in cyclohexane in a 250 ml beaker to yield a polymer concentration of 2% by weight.

- Heat mixture to the boiling point on a water bath to form a homogenous polymer solution.

- Take out the beaker from water bath and disperse the core material (ascorbic acid) in the solution with continuous stirring to get the coating to core material in the ratio of 1:2.

- Allow the mixture to cool with continuous stirring. It leads to phase separation coacervation of ethyl cellulose and microencapsulation of core material.

- Allow the mixture to further cool to room temperature for gelation and solidification of the coating.

- Collect the microencapsulated product from cyclohexane by filtration or decantation or centrifugation technique.

- Dry and weigh the product, and evaluate for following parameters.

Note: Compress the microcapsule of ascorbic acid in such a manner that each tablet has 50 mg of ascorbic acid. Determine the dissolution rate and compare it with plain ascorbic acid tablets (Experiment no. 6 and refer Table 6.2).

Evaluation

1. Organoleptic Properties

Color-

Odor-

Taste-

2. Size and Shape: By microscopic method.

3. % Yield: It is calculated by using following formula

% Yield = Practical yield/Theoretical yield × 100

4. Drug Content: Weigh the specific amount of the microcapsule powder. Dissolve in methanol and determine the amount of ascorbic acid spectrophometrically at λ_{max}......nm.

5. *In Vitro* Dissolution Studies: Perform in-vitro dissolution studies for microcapsules containing ascorbic acid by using dissolution apparatus one (Paddle type). Detail method is given in "Dissolution section". (Experiment no. 6 and refer Table 6.2).

Results:

1. Microcapsule was found to be spherical in shape.
2. Size of microcapsule was found to be _______ μm.
3. % yield of microcapsule was found to be _______ %.
4. After performing dissolution study, it was found that _______ % drug was released in _______ hours from microcapsules.

Precautions

1. Heating should be done on hot plate, avoid use of direct flame as cyclohexane is highly inflammable solvent.
2. Filtration of microparticles should be done with good quality filtration paper.
3. Microparticles should be dried in open air rather than by heating.

PHARMA TRIVIA: SELF EVALUATION TEST

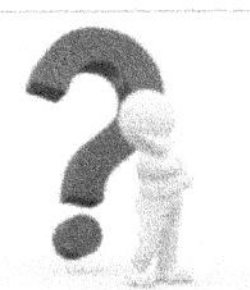

1. Define the term microencapsulation and write down its applications.

2. What are the various advantages and disadvantages of microencapsulation?

3. Name any two water soluble polymers.

4. Enlist various techniques used in encapsulation.

5. What are the various steps involved in phase separation coacervation method?

6. What is the ideal ratio of core: coat in phase separation coacervation method?

7. Explain briefly the air suspension method of microencapsulation.

8. Write down the principle of pan coating process.

9. Discuss briefly about the coating materials applicable in microencapsulation process.

10. Write the principle on incompatible polymer addition process.

11. Enumerate the various possible release mechanisms of microencapsulated product.

12. What are processing variables involved in air suspension?

13. Why microencapsulation is required for following drugs:
    (a) Vitamin A
    (b) Aspirin
    (c) Propranalol hydrochloride
    (d) Ascorbic acid

14. What are the various techniques used for phase separation coacervation.

15. Write down any two difference between spray drying and spray congealing.

7

Dispersed System

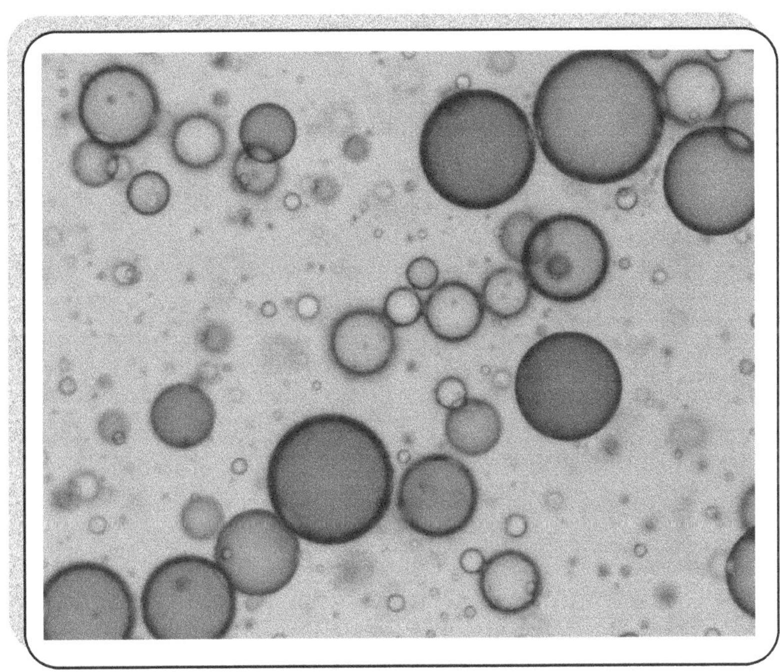

The term "Disperse System" refers to a heterogeneous kinetically stable and thermodynamically unstable biphasic or multiphase system. Basically in this system one phase known as the dispersed/internal phase is distributed, in the form of discrete units, throughout a second phase called continuous phase or vehicle or external phase. Disperse phase phase can exist in solid, liquid, or gaseous state while dispersion media may exist in the form of liquid or gas. Dispersed systems are divided into four types. They are

1. Coarse Dispersion (> 1 micron)
2. Colloidal Dispersion (1nm to 500 nm)
3. Fine Dispersion (500nm to 1 micron)
4. Solutions (< 1nm)

Suspensions and emulsions are coarse dispersed systems. A suspension is a biphasic solid -liquid, system in which insoluble solid particles (internal phase) of specific size range are dispersed evenly throughout the dispersion media with help of single or combination of suspending agents. The external phase (dispersion media) is generally aqueous but in some cases it may be combination of liquids, oils or purely organic solvents. While emulsions are biphasic liquid –liquid system in which dispersed phase is composed of small droplets of liquid distributed evenly throughout another liquid, with the help of single or combination of emulsifying agent.

Suspensions

Particles in a suspension are usually bigger than one micrometer and they are easily seen under a microscope and can often be seen with the naked eye. Particles in a suspension will always try to settle down (sediment) if the suspension is allowed to stand undisturbed due to the dominance of gravitational force. Rate of sedimentation is governed by stokes law. An examples of a simple suspension are chalk powder in water, or glass beads in water.

Applications

- To enhance the bioavailability of drug which is insoluble or poorly soluble E.g. Prednisolone suspension, Antacid suspension.
- Stability of some drugs is improved when they are given in insoluble form. E.g. Oxytetracycline suspension, Procaine penicillin G.

- To mask the objectionable or unpleasant or bitter taste drug. E.g. Chloramphenicol palmitate suspension and Paracetamol suspension
- Suspension of drug can be formulated in the form of lotion, paste and cream for various topical applications E.g. Calamine lotion, Zinc cream.
- Suspension can be formulated for parenteral controlled application and rate of drug absorption and duration can be controlled by varying the size of dispersed phase. E.g. Protamine Zinc-Insulin suspension, Cholera vaccine.
- Suspension can be used as a diagnosing agent. E.g. Barium sulphate suspension orally used as X-ray contrast agents for examination of GI tract discomfort.

Disadvantages of Suspensions

- Physical stability, sedimentation and wetting can causes problems.
- Relatively bulky so proper precaution must be taken during handling and transport.
- It is difficult to formulate
- Uniform and accurate dose cannot be achieved and hence potent drug cannot be given in this form.
- Preservation against the microbial contamination needs considerable attention.

Features of Ideal Pharmaceutical Suspensions

- Rate of particle sedimentation should be slow.
- If sediment forms, it should not form hard cake and must be easily re-suspended by gentle shaking
- Topical suspension should be free from gritty particles and having good spreadability.
- It should have pleasing organoleptic properties.
- Good pourability and syringeability.
- It should be physically and chemically stable during its shelf life..
- Should be resistant tomicrobiological contamination.
- Parenteral/Ophthalmic suspension should be sterilizable without compromising their stability.
- Should be free from cap-lock

Classification of Suspension

The suspension can be classified in various ways.

I.   Based on Route of Administration

   (i)   Oral suspension- e.g. Antacid Suspension

   (ii) Topical suspension-e.g.-Calamine lotion

   (iii) Parenteral suspension-e.g.Procaine Penicilline G

   (iv) Occular Suspension-e.g.Prednisolon, Brinzolamide

II.   Based on Dispersed Phase Content

   (i)   Dilute suspension (2 to10%w/v solid)

   (ii) Concentrated suspension (50%w/v solid)

III.   Based on Electrokinetic Nature of Solid Particles

   (i)   Flocculated suspension

   (ii) Deflocculated suspension

IV.   Based on Size of dispersed particles

   (i)   Colloidal suspension (< 1 micron)

   (ii) Coarse suspension (>1 micron)

   (iii) Molecular suspension (<1 nm)

Formulation Components

They are divided into two types:

   I.   Primary components and

   II. Secondary/Ancillary components

I.   Primary components: It includes

   1. Insoluble solids (Drug)

   2. Dispersion media

   3. Wetting agent

   4. Stabilizing agent: Suspending agent, Viscosity modifier, Flocculating agent etc

II.   Secondary/Ancillary components: It includes

   1. Buffering agent

   2. Preservatives

   3. Colouring agents

   4. Flavouring agents

Classification of Suspending Agents

I.   *Natural agents*: Tragacanth, Acacia Gum, Starch, Agar, Guar Gum, Carrageenan and Sodium Alginate.

II. *Semi-synthetic agents*: Hydroxyethylcellulose (Natrosol 250®), Sodium carboxymethylcellulose (Carmellose sodium®), Micro-crystalline cellulose (Avicel®).

III. *Synthetic agents*: Carbomer (Carboxyvinyl polymer, Carbopol®), Colloidal silicon dioxide (Aerosil®, Cab-o-sil®), Polyvinyl alcohol (PVA).

Suspending agents provide stability to the suspension by performing various mechanisms.

1.   Suspending agents form a thin film surrounding particles of dispersed phase and decrease interparticle attraction and hence minimize the aggregation which uiltimately reduce sedimentation. In addition suspending agents are also act as thickening/viscosifying agents and provide desired viscosity to the suspension, in order to avoid sedimentation of the suspended particles as well as formation of hard cake. It was observed that the suspension having a viscosity in the range of 200 -1500 milipoise is considered to be readily pourable suspension.

Ideally suspension should show thixotropic behaviour. At rest the suspension should have optimum viscosity to prevent aggregation and when shear (gentle shaking) is applied the viscosity is reduced and provide good pourability from the container. Xanthan gum, Carageenan, Na CMC/MCC, Avicel RC 591, Avicel RC 581 and Avicel CL 611 are some preferred suspending agents which provide thixotropic as well as pseudo-plastic behaviour.

Emulsions

Emulsion is defined as the thermodynamically unstable system of two immiscible liquids in which one liquid is dispersed in the form of small globules in another liquid which is the dispersion/continuous phase.

Classification of Emulsions:

I.   **Based on number of phase**

A. Biphasic emulsion

(a) Oil in Water (O/W): Oil droplets dispersed in water

(b) Water in Oil (W/O): Water droplets dispersed in oil

B. Multiphase emulsions

    (a) Oil-in-water-in-oil (O/W/O)

    (b) Water-in-oil-in-water (W/O/W)

II. Based on size of liquid droplets

    (a) Macroemulsions (Kinetically Stable) - 0.2 – 50 mm

    (b) Microemulsions (Thermodynamically Stable) – 20-200nm

    (c) Nanoemulsion (Kinetically Stable)- > 200nm

Factors affecting Type of Emulsion

- Type of emulsifying agent used
- Phase volume ratio
- Viscosity of each phase
- Shearing equipment
- Shearimg time

Applications of Emulsions

Emulsions are versatile dosage form and find a number of applications. Some important applications of emulsions are given below.

- *Topical delivery of drugs:* A large number of topical preparations including both medicated and nonmedicated are present in the form of lotions, creams and ointments which are mostly oil-in-water or water-in-oil type of emulsion as they are easily absorbed from the skin/mucosa. Several oily drugs are also given in the form emulsions to facilitate their absorption.

- *Bioavailability enhancement:* The oil soluble drugs are prepared in the form of o/w emulsion in order to improve the oral absorption and bioavailiability of poorly water-soluble drugs.

- *Sustained release of drug:* W/o emulsion can be used for sustained delivery of water soluble drugs.

- *Taste masking:* Simple and multiple emusions can be used for taste masking of several drugs

- *Drug delivery and targeting:* Emulsions can be given by different routes like oral, parenteral, topical, ocular etc. and hence they are versatile carriers for drugs and used in targeting of various drugs. The close similarities of fat emulsion particles to chylomicrons suggest that fat emulsions can be used as carrier for drugs and as targeted delivery systems to lymph.

- *Parenteral nutritional supplements:* A major application of lipid emulsions is the delivery of fat in parenteral nutrition. Fat is a strong source of energy and can supply essential fatty acids. Digestion of fats in the intestine is facilitated by o/w emulsion

- *Stability:* Emulsions especially o/w can enhance the stability of certain drugs by providing a non-aqueous environment. Many drugs, like barbituric acid, diazepam, and anesthetics are prone to hydrolytic degradation, have been dissolved in the oil phase (o/w emulsion) and administered by all types of parenteral routes.

Formulation Components

I.   **Primary components:** It includes
   1. Dispersed /Internal/Discontinuous phase
   2. Dispersion/External/Continuous phase
   3. Stabilizing agent (Emulsifying agent)

II. **Secondary/Ancillary components:** It includes
   1. Buffering agent
   2. Organoleptic agents- Colouring, Flavouring and Sweetening agent
   3. Preservatives

Preparation of Emulsions

Emulsions on large scale are usually prepared by vigorously mixing the two immiscible liquids by mechanically using either a high speed mixers or by using ultrasonicator. While on laboratory scale they are generally prepared manually by using simple pestle mortar. This process is known as emulsification. Since these two liquids are completely immiscible, a stabilizing agent, known as emulsifying agent or emulsifier of a particular HLB value is used in continuous phase to stabilize the resulting emulsion. The emulsifiers with higher HLB value (8-16) are used in o/w emulsion preparation while low HLB emulsifier used in w/o emulsion preparation.

In the absence of emulsifying agent, the dispersed phase globules coalesce together to form larger globules which ultimately lead to breaking up of emulsion into two separate layers. Some of the important emulsifying agents used in pharmaceutical industries are soaps, proteins, gums, Spans, Tweens and lecithin. Among these, soaps and detergents are most commonly used emulsifiers.

Role of Emulsifier

The emulsifying agent forms a protective film around the oil droplets dispersed in water. This layer prevents them to come closer and to coalesce, i.e. to combine together. Thus, the emulsion gets stabilized. For example, when sodium lauryl sulphate is added to an o/w emulsion, the molecules arrange themselves in such a way that the polar end groups immerse in water whereas the hydrocarbon chains dip in oil droplet as shown in the figure below. Thus hydrophilic molecules get concentrated over the surface of the oil droplet and form a protective film. This decreases the interfacial tension between oil and water and aggregation among the droplets hence emulsion gets stabilized.

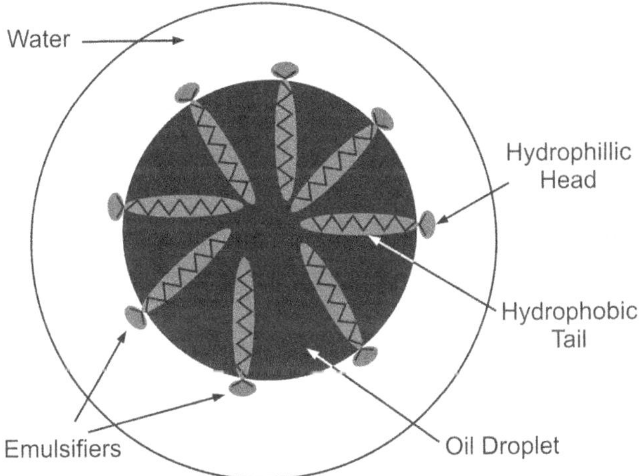

Arrangement of emulsifier in oil in water emulsion

Emulsifying agent can be cationic, anionic, nonionic and amphoteric. based on the charge they carry. Nonionic surfactants like spans and tweens are mostly used in pharmaceutical preparation due to their inert nature. Based on their source they can be classified into natural, synthetic or semisynthetic.

Identification of Emulsion Type

The type of an emulsion can be determined by performing any of the following tests.

- ***Dilution test:*** In this test few drops of water is added to the given emulsion. If the added water mixes completely with the emulsion, the emulsion is of oil-in-water (o/w) type. In case the added water does not mix up with the emulsion, the given emulsion is of water-in-oil (w/o) type. Similarly if the emulsion on dilution with oil remains stable then it is a w/o emusion

- *Conductivity test:* This test involves the addition of a small amount of electrolyte to the emulsion under the examination followed by the measurement of its conductance. If the conductance increases, the emulsion is of oil-in-water type as water is a good conductor of electricity and if there is no significant change in the conductance, the emulsion is of water-in-oil type.

- *Dye test:* In this test, a small amount of an oil-soluble dye is added to the emulsion. If the emulsion becomes coloured, it is of water-in-oil type. If no change in colour is observed, the emulsion is of oil-in-water type.

- *Fluoroscence test:* Since certain oils show fluorescence under UV light. O/W emulsion exhibits dot pattern while w/o emulsion shows fluoresce throughout.

- *Cobalt chloride test:* Impregnate filter paper with Cocl2 solution and dry, paper becomes blue Now put some drops of o/w emulsion color changes to pink

- *Bancroft rule:* This rule states that type of emulsion will be governed by relative solubility of emulsifier. The phase in which it is more soluble being the dispersion media (continuous phase). For example Emulsion having 1:1 water and oil ratio and contains water soluble surfactant, o/w emulsion will form

Properties of Emulsions

The size of the dispersed phase droplets in emulsions may be somewhat larger as compared to the size of dispersed particles in solutions. Still, emulsions are colloidal systems and exhibit all the properties exhibited by colloidal solutions e.g. Brownian movement, Tyndall effect, electrophoresis, coagulation etc.

Emulsions are prone towards physical and chemical degradation. They can be broken into their constituent liquids either by physical methods such as heating, freezing, centrifuging etc. or by chemical method such as degradation of the emulsifying agent The process of breaking an emulsion to yield the constituent liquids is called demulsification.

Emulsification Equipments

1. *Small scale:* Pestle and mortar, shaker
2. *Large scale:* Turbines, colloid mill, Propeller, Homogenizer, Uitrasonicator, Microfludizer etc

Methods of preparation: Emulsions are prepared by following methods

1. Dry gum or continental method
2. Wet gum method
3. Beaker method
4. Bottle or Forbes bottle method
5. Phase Inversion method
6. Mcmbrane emulsification method

Characterization of Dispersed Systems

The dispersed systems are characterized for various parameters. These parameters are evaluated in freshly prepared as well as stored dispersed systems. Minimum change in the value indicates the good stability of system. The parameters include-colour, odour, pH, density, viscosity, particle/globule size, Sedimentation rate and ratio (for suspension), creaming cracking, phase separation (for emulsion), drug release, drug content, dissolution study and rate of permeation across the skin or mucosa.

23

To Prepare and Evaluate Three Antacid Suspensions and Compare their Stability

Requirements: Pestle mortar, measuring cylinders (3), excipients, pH paper, density bottle, viscometer, microscope

Reference: Refer any book given in the list of books at the beginning of this manual.

Formula

S. No.	Ingredients	Formula 1	Formula 2	Formula 3
1.	Aluminium hydroxide	23.3 g	23.3 g	23.3 g
2.	Magnesium hydroxide	13.11 g	13.11 g	13.11
3.	Potassium citrate	-	0.6 g	-
4.	Sorbitol (70%)	-	-	10.0 g
5.	Methyl paraben	0.2 g	0.2 g	0.2 g
6.	Propyl paraben	0.02 g	0.02 g	0.02 g
7.	Saccharin	0.1 g	0.1 g	0.1 g
8.	Peppermint oil	0.005	0.005	0.005
9.	Alcohol	1 ml	1 ml	1 ml
10.	Purified water	100 ml	100 ml	100 ml

Principle

Suspensions are the heterogeneous systems consisting of two phases. The continuous or the external phase generally a liquid or semisolid and the dispersed or internal phase is made up of particulate matter that is essentially insoluble in, but dispersed throughout the continuous phase. The dispersed phase may consist of discrete particle or the network of the particles resulting from particle-particle interactions. An ideal suspension must remain sufficiently homogeneous for at least the period of time necessary to remove and administer the required dose after shaking its container. The suspensions are usually prepared by dispersion method or precipitation method.

Antacid constitutes a single class of drugs available in both tablet and suspension forms. However, the suspensions are much more effective and quicker in onset as they spread well in surface as there is disintegration lag time. The present formulation is prepared by dispersion method. Aluminium hydroxide and magnesium hydroxide have antacid (pH rising) effect. Aluminium hydroxide (but not magnesium hydroxide) antacid suspension has a tendency to thicken during shelf life and further aluminium hydroxide has a constipating effect. Therefore magnesium hydroxide is used in present formulation to impart the laxative effect. Potassium citrate (anti-gelling agent) is also added to the system to reduce thickening of aluminium hydroxide. Methyl paraben and propyl paraben are used as preservative along with alcohol. Peppermint oil, saccharin and sorbitol are used to enhance the taste and palatability of the formulation.

The techniques for the evaluation of heterogeneous systems are generally complex and are far from being completely satisfactory. Commonly used methods for the evaluation includes sedimentation techniques, rheological techniques, electro-kinetic techniques and micromeritic techniques.

Procedure

- Dissolve the methyl paraben, propylparaben, saccharin and peppermint oil in alcohol.
- Transfer the mixture with agitation to a vessel containing nearly one half of the volume of purified water in which either potassium citrate or sorbitol has been dissolved **(Formula 2 and 3).**
- Place the weighed quantity of aluminium hydroxide and magnesium hydroxide powder in a pestle and mortar.
- Triturate this powder with the aqueous solution prepared in step two until the smooth paste is obtained.
- Add the remaining purified water with the continuous stirring and adjust the final volume.

Note: Use same method for preparation of antacid suspension without taking potassium citrate or sorbitol (Formula 1).

Evaluation of Suspension: The formulation is evaluated for following parameters

A. **Organoleptic Evaluation:** Under this, suspension is evaluated for following parameters

   1. Color

   2. Taste (For oral suspension only)

   3. Odor

B. **Sedimentation Method:** Physical stability is defined as the condition in which the particles remain uniformly distributed throughout the dispersion without any sign of sedimentation. It is difficult to achieve this condition. Hence the definition can be restated as if the particles settle, they should be easily resuspendable by a moderate amount of shaking. Therefore the extent of sedimentation and ease of redispersibility are to be evaluated by appropriate method.

The extent of sedimentation is quantitatively expressed by following parameters.

   1. Sedimentation Ratio

   2. Rate of sedimentation

   3. Degree of flocculation

      1. Sedimentation Ratio: It is denoted by following formula

$$F = \frac{H_u}{H_o} = \frac{\text{Ultimate height of sediment}}{\text{Initial height of suspension}}$$

F is denoted as sedimentation ratio or sedimentation volume, it is a dimensionless number

When $F = 1$ i.e., $H_u = H_o$, is a desirable properly of an ideal suspension.

On the contrary

   $F = 0$, i.e., $H_u = 0$ indicates total instability

Normally F value is between 0 to 1. In general the higher the sedimentation ratio, the better is the physical stability.

Sedimentation ratio generally varies with time. When plotted against time abscissa, it gives a curve that indicates the sedimentation pattern on storage. If the curve is horizontal to time axis it indicates a better suspension. However, if it steeps down it indicates a poor formulation.

Method: Keep a measured volume (H_o) of the suspension in a graduated cylinder/tube in an undisturbed state for a certain period of time and note the volume of sediment (H_u) at various time intervals. Calculate sedimentation ratio at each time interval and plot a curve between sedimentation ratio and time.

2. **Rate of Sedimentation:** It can be described by Stokes law which gives the velocity, v, of a spherical particle (radius r and density σ) falling in a liquid of density ρ and viscosity η where g is the acceleration due to gravity. Theoretically it is expressed by

$$v = 2a^2g(\sigma - \rho)/9\eta$$

In laboratory it is calculated by

$$R = \frac{H}{t} = \frac{\text{Height of sediment at time t}}{\text{Time}}$$

Method: Note height of sediment in the method described above and calculates sedimentation rate by dividing height of sediment with time elapsed.

3. **Degree of Flocculation (β):** It is defined as ratio of volume of sediment to the volume of total dispersion and it is given by the following formula:

$$\beta = \frac{F}{F_\alpha}$$

where

F = sedimentation ratio of flocculated system (H_u)

$$\text{i.e., } = \frac{F}{H_o} = \frac{H_u}{H_o}$$

F_α= sedimentation ratio of deflocculated system ($F_\alpha = H_\alpha$)

$$\text{i.e., } \frac{F_\alpha}{H_o} = \frac{H_\alpha}{H_o}$$

$$\beta = \frac{H_u/H_o}{H_\alpha/H_0} = \frac{H_u}{H_\alpha}$$

$$\beta = \frac{\text{Ultimate height of sediment in flocculated system } H_u}{\text{Ultimate height of sediment in deflocculated system } H_\alpha}$$

C. **Particle Size:** Any change in particle size with reference to time will give useful information regarding the stability of a suspension. A change in particle size distribution may be studied by microscopic method or by coulter counter method or by Andreasen pipette method.

   Method: In the microscopic method first calibrate ocular micrometer with the help of stage micrometer and calculate least count. Put a drop of diluted suspension on a slide and spread to form a thin film. Put a cover slip and note the number of particles falling under the divisions of micrometer. Total particles counted should at least be 500. Arithmetic mean of these measurements is taken as measure of particle size.

D. **Electro Kinetic Method:** Surface electric charged or zeta potential is an important factor affecting stability of the suspensions. Measurement of zeta potential is done on the basis of electrophoretic velocity of the particles. The instrument used for this purpose is zeta meter. In this instrument, electric field is created by application of voltage between electrodes. Sample of the suspension is placed in the electric field so created and consequent mobility of several particles of suspension is measured. Zeta potential is calculated as under:

$$\mathbf{Z_P \text{ (in mV)} = 4\pi nu / \xi E}$$

   where

       n = Viscosity of dispersion media in poise

       u = Average migration velocity of particles in cm/s

       E = Potential gradient

          (voltage applied/distance between electrodes)

       ξ = Dielectric constant of dispersion media

E. **Rheological Method:** Rheological behavior of the suspension helps to know about stability of the suspension. This essentially involves viscosity measurement by Brookfield viscometer.

This instrument comes with several spindles. The sample is sheared for a particular time using appropriate spindle. Reading of the indicator dial is taken.

F. **Ease of Redispersibility (Content Uniformity):** It is the uniformity of suspended drug dosage delivered from a suspension product, from the first volumetric dose out of the bottle to the last, under one or more standard shaking conditions as just described below.

    Method: Shake the suspension with the help of a mechanical device, which simulates motion of human arm during shaking (manually shake the suspension at-least 10 times). Measure the drug content in 5 ml of suspension by prescribed method (UV spectrophotometric method/ titration method/etc). Repeat the experiment 3 times; if drug content is same every time, it indicates redispersibility of suspension and uniformity of dose.

G. **pH Determination:** Determine the pH by pH paper or by pH meter.

H. **Density:** Take weight of dry empty density bottle. Fill bottle with distilled water and weigh. Fill the bottle with prepared suspension and weigh it again.

Observations

1. Weight of dry empty density bottle= w1
2. Weight of dry empty density bottle + water = w2
3. Weight of dry empty density bottle + suspension= w3

Calculation

Density of Suspension = Weight of suspension (w3 – w1)/Weight of water (w2 – w1)

Observation Table

S. No.	Parameters	Formula 1		Formula 2		Formula 3		Inference
		Fresh	After 1 week	Fresh	After 1 week	Fresh	After 1 week	
1.	Color							
2.	Odor							
3.	pH							
4.	Particle Size							
5.	Sedimentation Ratio							

Table *Contd...*

S. No.	Parameters	Formula 1		Formula 2		Formula 3		Inference
		Fresh	After 1 week	Fresh	After 1 week	Fresh	After 1 week	
6.	Sedimentation Rate							
7.	Viscosity							
8.	Density							
9.	Zeta-potential							
10.	Drug Content							

Results: Three different antacid suspensions were prepared and evaluated for different parameters.

24

To Prepare Liquid Paraffin Emulsion I.P. and Determine the Effect of Homogenization Time on Globule Size Distribution

Requirements: Pestle mortar, mixer (magnetic stirrer/homogenizer/mechanical stirrer) microscope, stage & ocular micrometer, glass slide, cover slip, excipients.

Reference: Refer any book given in the list of books at the beginning of this manual.

Formula

S. No.	Ingredients	Quantity Given	Quantity Taken
1.	Heavy liquid Paraffin	50 ml	
2.	Span 80	2.52 ml	
3.	Tween 80	3.48 ml	
4.	Sodium benzoate	0.5 g	
5.	Vanilin	0.05 g	
6.	Glycerin	12.5 ml	
7.	Chloroform	0.25 ml	
8.	Water (q.s.)	50.0 ml	

Principle

An emulsion is a system consisting of two immiscible liquid phases, one of which is dispersed throughout the other in the form of fine droplets. A third component, the emulsifying agent is necessary to stabilize the emulsion. Emulsifying agent surrounding the droplets of internal phase as a thin layer of film adsorbed on the surface of the droplets and prevents their contact and coalescence. The phase that is present as fine droplets is called the disperse phase and the phase in which the droplets are suspended is the continuous phase. Depending on the nature of dispersed phase and dispersion medium, the emulsion can be classified as water in oil (W/O) or oil in water (O/W). The emulsifying agent of low HLB value (3-6) are used for the preparation of W/O emulsions while emulsifying agents with the higher HLB values (8-18) are used for the preparation of O/W emulsion. More complicated emulsion systems may exist: for example, an oil droplet enclosing a water droplet may be suspended in water to form a water-in-oil-in water emulsion (w/o/w). Such systems or their o/w/o counterparts are termed as multiple emulsions and are of interest as delayed-action drug delivery systems.

Various equipments are used for the mixing of the two phases (emulsification) such as pestle mortar (small scale), overhead stirrer, magnetic stirrer, blender and homogenizer. The shear force and time for shearing are the two important parameters in the formation of stable and uniform globule size.

In the present experiment, an O/W emulsion is prepared by using liquid paraffin as oil phase and span-80 and tween-80 as emulsifying agents. Vanillin and chloroform are used as flavoring agents. Sodium benzoate and chloroform are used as preservatives. Glycerin is used as viscosity enhancing agent.

Procedure

- Mix span 80 and tween 80 in oil (50 ml) and water (35 ml) respectively.

- Add liquid paraffin phase (oily phase) to the aqueous phase little by little with continuous stirring in a pestle mortar or by magnetic stirrer/ mechanical stirrer.

- Add sodium benzoate, vanillin and glycerin to the water (5 ml) and then add it to the emulsion with continuous stirring. Make up volume 100 ml with water.

- Stir the emulsion continuously for five minutes to stabilize the emulsion.

- Withdraw 1 ml samples at 0, 2, 4, 6, 8 and 10 minutes time interval into the test tubes by stopping the mixer each time.

- Dilute each sample to 10 ml with water and determine the globule size and size distribution.

Determination of globule size and size distribution:

1. Take a drop of dilute emulsion from each sample and prepare a slide.
2. Count diameters of 100 globules from 5 different positions by microscopic method.
3. Plot a graph between the number of globules on Y axis and globule size range on X-axis.

Note: Emulsification can be done by trituration (low shear technique) or by magnetic stirrer/mechanical stirrer/sonication/homogeniser (according to availability of equipment).

Observations and Calculations

No. of divisions on stage micrometer = divisions of occulomicrometer

No. of divisions on occulomicrometer =

100 divisions of stage micrometer =

1 division of stage micrometer =

Thus 1 division of occulomicrometer =

Observation Table

S. No.	Range	Mean globule size (d)	No. of particles (n)	nd	nd^2
1.	0-10				
2.	10-20				
3.	20-30				
4.	30-40				
5.	40-50				

$$\Sigma n = \Sigma nd, \Sigma nd^2$$

Calculate mean surface diameter (d_s) by the following formula:

$$ds = \sqrt{\Sigma nd^2 / \Sigma n}$$

S. No.	Time for Homogenization (Minutes)	Surface Diameter (dsn)
1.	2	
2.	4	
3.	6	
4.	8	
5.	10	

Results: The droplet size of emulsion was found to be decreased with increase in homogenization time.

25

To Determine the HLB of Liquid Paraffin Using Modified Gum Acacia Method

Requirements: Pestle mortar, 6 measuring cylinders, pipette, acacia, tween 80, liquid paraffin, distilled Water.

Reference: Refer any book given in the list of books at the beginning of this manual.

Formula

S. No.	Ingredients	Quantity given	Quantity taken
1.	Liquid paraffin	15 ml	
2.	Mixture of gum acacia and Tween 80	5 g	
3.	Water q.s.	100 ml	

Principle

The **Hydrophilic-lipophilic balance** of a surfactant is a measure of the degree to which it is hydrophilic or lipophilic, and determined by calculating values for the different regions of the molecule, as described by Griffin in 1949 and 1954.

The HLB value can be used to predict the surfactant properties:

- A value from 1 to 3 indicates an anti-foaming agent
- A value from 3 to 8 indicates a W/O (water in oil) emulsifier
- A value from 7 to 9 indicates a wetting agent

- A value from 8 to 16 indicates O/W (oil in water) emulsifier
- A value from 13 to 16 indicates a detergent
- A value of 16 to 18 indicates a solubilizer

The HLB of a number of polyhydric alcohol fatty acid esters, such as glyceryl monostearate may be estimated by the following formula:

$$\textbf{HLB} = \textbf{20 (1 – S/A)}$$

where, S is the saponification number of the ester and A the acid number of the fatty acid.

Davies has calculated HLB values for surface-active agents by splitting the various surfactant molecules into their component groups, each of which is assigned a group number. Summation of the respective group numbers for a particular surfactant permits calculation of its HLB value according to the following equation:

$$HLB = 7 + \Sigma H_i - 0.475 \times n$$

where H_i is Value of ith Hydrophilic group

n is Number of lipophilic groups in the molecule

Approximations of the HLB for surfactants whose HLB is not defined by Griffin or Davies system, can be determined by either from their water dispersibility or from an experimental estimation of their HLBs. Blends of the unknown emulsifier in varying ratios with an emulsifier of known HLB are used to emulsify an oil of known "required" HLB. The blend that performs best (negligible phase separation) is assumed to have an HLB value approximately equal to the "required" HLB of the oil. The required HLB can be calculated by the following formula

$$\text{Required HLB of liquid paraffin} = \frac{W_A HLB_A + W_B HLB_B}{W_A + W_B}$$

where

HLB_A = HLB of first surfactant

HLB_B = HLB of second surfactant

W_A = Weight of First surfactant

W_B = Weight of second surfactant

Note: In the present experiment liquid paraffin is used as an oil phase and Tween 80 (HLB = 15) and gum acacia (HLB = 8) are used as surfactant.

Procedure

- Prepare a series of six emulsions by taking different ratio of acacia and tween 80.
- Take liquid paraffin (15 ml) as the dispersed phase and water as the dispersion medium.
- A mixture of gum acacia and tween 80 (ratio is given in observation table) is used as the emulsifying agent.
- Take emulsifying agent in a dry mortar and make into a solution with small quantity of warm water.
- Add liquid paraffin slowly and a little at time along with trituration.
- Continue triluratation till whole of liquid paraffin is incorporated.
- Make the volume to 100 ml in a measuring cylinder.
- Repeat same method for different ratios and prepare total six emulsions and keep into a measuring cylinder for 24 hours.
- The formulation which shows minimum height of creaming, shows maximum stability and considered for final HLB calculation for the formulation.
- Note the height/volume of creaming for each emulsion.

Observation table

S. No.	Weight of Acacia (A) (g)	Weight of Tween 80 (B) (g)	Required HLB* (calculated value)	Height/Volume of creaming (cm/ml)	Inference
1.	0	5			
2.	1	4			
3.	2	3			
4.	3	2			
5.	4	1			
6.	5	0			

$$\text{*Required HLB of liquid paraffin} = \frac{W_A HLB_A + W_B HLB_B}{W_A + W_B}$$

where

HLB_A = HLB of acacia 8

HLB_B = HLB of Tween 80, 15

W_A = Weight of Acacia at maximum stability

W_B = Weight of Tween 80 at maximum stability

Results: HLB of liquid paraffin in o/w emulsion calculated by modified gum acacia method was found to be _______.

PHARMA TRIVIA: SELF EVALUATION TEST

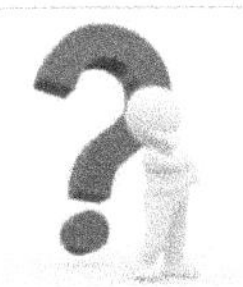

1. What are the various tests to identify the type of emulsion?
2. What is the difference between flocculated and deflocculated suspension?
3. What factor distinguishes a suspension from a colloid?
4. What are emulsions? How are they classified?
5. How do you differentiate O/W and W/O type of emulsion?
6. Describe the Bancroft Rule.
7. What is the importance of HLB Scale?
8. Write two examples of an emulsifying agent used in preparation of w/o emulsion
9. Write the formula for liquid paraffin emulsion IP.
10. Differentiate between creaming and cracking of emulsions.
11. Explain the stability of emulsions.
12. List out the advantages of emulsions.
13. List out the applications of suspensions.
14. Mention the various characterization parameters for emulsion.
15. Mention the various characterization parameters for suspension.

8

Aerosol

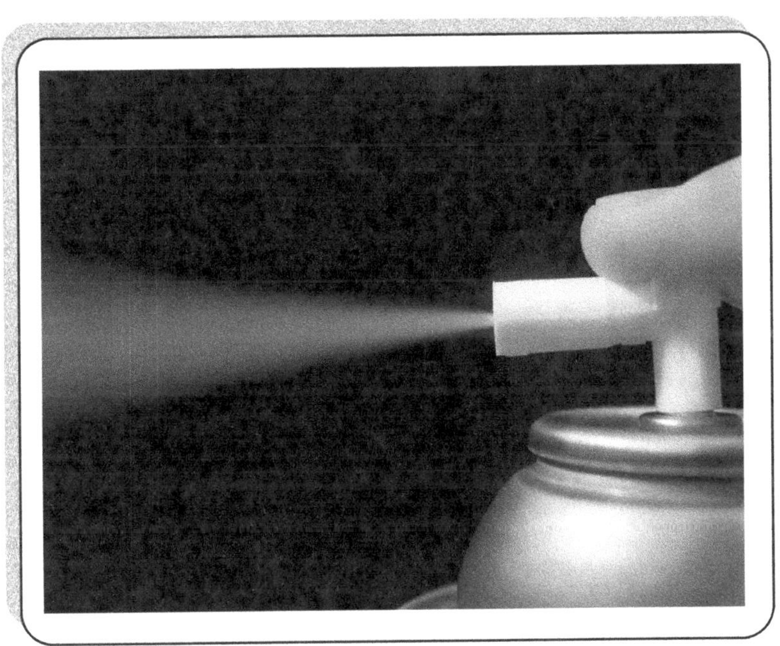

The term "Aerosol" is used to denote various types of systems ranging from those having a colloidal nature to systems which consist of pressurized packages. Aerosol, as suggested by its name, can be simply defined as a dispersed phase system in which very fine particles of solid drug or fine droplets of liquid are dispersed in a gaseous continuous phase known as propellants. An Aerosol system is a system designed to expel the contents from the container that depends on the pressure developed by the compressed or liquefied gas. Aerosols can also be simply understood as dispersions in which dispersed phase is either solid or liquid and continuous phase is a gas (propellants).

Pharmaceutical aerosols may therefore be defined as aerosol formulations which contain therapeutically active agents, either dissolved, suspended or emulufied with a propellant (or a mixture of propellants) meant for administration into body cavities such as ear, rectum. But more commonly, they are intended to be administered through oral or nasal route as fine solid suspended particles or liquid mists to be absorbed through the respiratory system, nasal passages or sublingual route.

So basically, an aerosol is a pressurized dosage form which contains one or more active ingredients and releases a fine dispersion (particles smaller than 50 μm) of liquid and/or solid materials in a gaseous medium. This gives an aerosol its other names such as Pressurized Packages, Pressure Package or Pressurized dosage forms. Pressure is developed in the aerosol system by using one or more liquefied or gaseous propellants.

Advantages

Aerosol dosage form offers a number of advantages:

1. First advantage of aerosols is that they successfully avoid any kind of contamination. As they have a closed packing, there is no manual/direct contact with the medicament while administering. Required quantity of medicament is conveniently withdrawn from the aerosol system without contaminating the remaining medicament.

2. Second advantage is the accurate dosing. Specific amount of medicament can be delivered by pressing the metered valve. With

the help of metered valves, the same amount of drug is released every time. This also maintains the uniformity of the dosing.

3. Since the dosing is uniform and administration is very simple, the drug can be easily and conveniently self-administered by the patient without taking help from anybody else. This improves the patient compliance.

4. As compared to other dosage forms, aerosols are preferred choice for targeting as they deliver the drug directly to the affected area.

5. Aerosols lead to faster onset of action.

6. Since the drug is directly delivered to the target site, it by passes the first pass metabolism.

7. This route of drug administration also helps in avoiding decomposition or inactivation of drug by the pH or enzymatic action of the stomach or intestine.

8. Few drugs are sensitive to the atmospheric oxygen or moisture and are destabilized when exposed. This makes their administration a challenge. But with aerosols, stability of these drugs does not pose any problem as the drug is not exposed to the atmosphere and is directly delivered into the body. Also, drug remains stable inside the container as well because the propellant inside does not contain any water, neither any oxygen is present.

9. Similarly, sterility can be maintained for sterile formulations as microorganisms cannot enter the container even when the valve is open.

10. As the aerosol containers do not allow even light to enter, they are ideal for photosensitive drugs also and protect them from decomposition due to light.

11. Aerosols are ideal for administration through nasal route by inhalation as the drug is delivered in the form of a fine mist. Fine mist is rapidly volatilized which leaves a cooling, refreshing effect.

12. Sprays and foams applied topically to the skin reduce or eliminate the irritation brought about by mechanical application of medication to abraded areas of the skin.

13. Dose can be tailored to suit individual needs and ideal for 'prn' medications (use when necessary).

14. Aerosols serve as viable alternative when the drug entity exhibits erratic pharmacokinetics upon oral or parenteral administration.

15. Aerosols present themselves as a more efficient dosage form as there is no wastage or messy administration (such as use of cotton swabs, applicator).

Disadvantages

Though highly advantageous, aerosols possess few disadvantages too. They are:

1. Firstly, in order to formulate a drug as an aerosol, the drug must be soluble in the propellant.
2. Aerosols are not pocket friendly and are comparatively more expensive.
3. Disposal of empty aerosol containers is also an environmental issue.
4. Occasionally, the propellants might irritate the injured skin due to their volatile nature.
5. Continuous use of aerosol for a long duration, few propellants may cause toxic reactions. Some patients may be sensitive and allergic towards propellants and use of aerosols is not advisable for them.
6. In case of inhalation aerosols, the fluorinated hydrocarbons may cause carcinogenic effects on prolonged usage.
7. Most importantly, all the aerosols must be kept away from fire and high temperature conditions as they may develop high pressure inside the container which can leads to explosion.

Components of Aerosol Package

Following are the four main components of an aerosol system:

1. Propellants
2. container
3. Valve and actuators
4. Product concentrates

Types of Aerosols

Aerosols are basically of following types:

1. Two phase systems or solution system (Vapor and Liquid)
2. Three phase systems or Water based systems (Gas, Liquid and Solid/Liquid)
3. Foam aerosols or Emulsion system

1. Two phase systems (Gas and liquid)

These aerosols contain two phases, that is, liquid phase and gas phase. Gas phase is always comprised of vapors of the liquefied propellant. And here, the liquid phase is the liquefied propellant in which the solution of the active ingredients is mixed. This liquid phase may also contain other liquids such as co solvents like alcohols, glycols etc. The point here is that all the ingredients are miscible with each other, are in liquid state and there are no solid particles.

2. Three phase systems (Gas, Liquid and Solid/Liquid)

With increased emphasis upon the decrease of volatile oil organic compounds (VOCS) in all products these systems are finding increased use. Large amount of water can be used to replace all or part of the non aqueous solvents used in aerosols. This system is composed of a layer of water immiscible liquid propellant, highly aqueous product concentrate and the vapor phase. This type of system employed when the product is immiscible with the propellant. Ethanol used as a co-solvent to solubilize propellant in the water.

3. Foam Aerosols

Foam aerosols are typically emulsions composed of the active ingredients, surfactants, propellants and other aqueous or non-aqueous liquids. If propellant (non-aqueous liquid) is the dispersed phase, i.e. the emulsion is of oil-in-water type, the aerosol is discharged in the form of stable foam. And if the propellant is the continuous phase, i.e. the emulsion is of water-in-oil type, the aerosol is discharged in the form of a spray or quick-breaking foam.

Working of Aerosols

As already stated, aerosols are the dispersions where fine solid particles or liquid droplets are dispersed in liquefied gas propellant or a mixture of propellants. This dispersion is sealed in an aerosol container. Inside the container, the propellant is continuously evaporating. Very soon, the evaporation reaches the stage of equilibrium where the liquefied propellant and the vapors of the propellant exist in equilibrium inside the container.

At this equilibrium state, the vapor phase exerts a specific pressure on the walls of the container, at the valve assembly, and at the surface of the liquid phase which contains the liquefied propellant and the drug. This pressure results in the actuation of the aerosol valve and forces the liquid phase to the dip tube and through the orifice of the valve. This ultimately causes the release of the liquid from the orifice into the atmosphere. When the propellant is released into the atmosphere, it faces a sharp drop in the pressure because of which it expands and evaporates. This converts the liquid into airborne droplets or dry particles, as the type of the formulation may be. In addition to the formulation type, the physical state of the contents emitted also depends on the type of valve used. Usually, aerosol containers are designed to release their contents in the form of a fine mist or a dry spray.

When a portion of the liquid phase is withdrawn from the container, equilibrium again gets established between the remaining amounts of propellant and its vapors. Therefore, the pressure inside the container remains constant even during the expulsion, and the formulation is continuously released in the same proportion and at the same rate. The pressure cannot be maintained only when the liquid reservoir is completely depleted.

Manufacture of Pharmaceutical Aerosols

Following are the apparatus that are used for the manufacture of aerosols:

1. Pressure filling apparatus
2. Cold filling apparatus
3. Compressed gas-filling apparatus.

Manufacturing procedures generally takes place in two stages. They are

Stage I: Manufacture of concentrate

Stage II: Addition of propellant

Quality Control for Pharmaceutical Aerosols

1. *Propellant:* Propellants are tested for the following attributes:
   (i) Density
   (ii) Vapor pressure
   (iii) Purity
   (iv) Identity (by gas chromatography)
   (v) Composition (by gas chromatography), when a mixture of different propellants is used

2. ***Valves actuators and dip tubes:*** Valves Actuators and Dip tubes are subjected to physical as well as chemical inspection:

   (i) Inertness.

   (ii) Physical stability: Softening, cracking, elongation or distortion

3. ***Containers:*** Containers are examined for:

   (a) Dip elongation and cracking

   (b) Defects in lining.

   (c) Glass container examined for any kind of flaws.

   (d) Dimensions of all the parts such as neck. All dimensions must conform to specifications.

   (e) Weight

4. ***Weight checking:*** This method consists of

   (a) Periodically adding to filling line tarred empty aerosol containers, which after being filled with concentrate, are removed and weighed.

   (b) The similar procedure is used to check the weight of propellant that is being added.

   (c) The finished container is weighed for further accuracy of the filling operation.

Leak testing: It consists of checking the crimping of the valve in order to check any leakage from the container. It involves following steps-

(a) Pass the filled container through the water bath.

(b) Periodic checks are made of the temperature of the water bath and results are recorded. If any air bubbles are seen in water bath indicates the leakage from the container

(c) D.O.T. (Department of transportation)-According to this "each completed container filled for shipment must have been heated until contents reached a minimum of 130^0F.

Spray testing: This test is used to check any defects in valve and spray pattern.

Evaluation of Pharmaceutical Aerosols

1. **Flammability and Combustibility**

   I. ***Flash point:*** Flash point is estimated by the standard "Tag open Cup Apparatus".

Method: To perform this test, the aerosol product is cooled down to a temperature of –25°F and then it is transferred to the test apparatus. The temperature of the test liquid is then allowed to increase gradually, and the temperature at which the ignition of vapors takes place is recorded as the flash point.

II. *Flame extension:* This test is performed to determine the effect of the aerosol formulation on the extension of an open flame.

Method: The aerosol product is sprayed into a flame for a short duration of 4 seconds. The flame gets extended according to the nature of the formulation. The exact length of the flame extension is then measured with a scale.

2. Physiochemical Characteristics

I. *Vapor pressure:* The pressure can be measured through a pressure gauge or by using a water bath, test gauges and other special equipment. Large variations in the values among containers indicate towards the presence of air in the headspace.

II. *Density:* The density of an aerosol system can be measured by hydrometer or a pycnometer.

III. *Moisture content:* It can be determined either by gas chromatography or by Karl Fischer method.

IV. *Identification of propellant and concentrate-propellant ratio:* Gas chromatography and infra-red spectrophotometric methods are used for identification and determination of proportion of each component in a blend.

3. Performance

I. *Aerosol valve discharge rate:*

Method: Determine the weight of the aerosol container, discharge the content for given period of time and then reweigh the container. Difference in weight /time (gm/sec) gives the rate of discharge.

II. *Spray patterns:* This test is based on the impingement of the spray on a piece of paper which has previously been treated with a mixture of dye and talc. Dye can be oil-soluble or water-soluble, depending on the nature of the aerosol. The striking of aerosol particles with the paper results in absorption of the dye into the paper. This gives a spray record which can be used for comparisons.

III. *Dosage with metered valves:* This is done in order to check the **reproducibility of dosage** each time the valve is depressed and to calculate the **amount of medication** actually received by the patient.

Method I: This is based on assay technique. One or two doses are to be dispensed into a solvent or onto a material that absorbs the active ingredients. The assay of the solvent or the adsorbent material is then performed to determine the amount of the active ingredients.

Method II: In this method, filled container is weighed accurately and then several doses are dispensed. The container is weighed again and the difference in weight is divided by the number of doses dispensed to give the average dose.

IV. *Net contents:* The test is performed to check whether required quantity of product has been placed in each container. For this, first weigh the empty aerosol container and after filling the product reweigh the container. Difference in weight will give the net content.

V. *Foam stability:* Foam can remain stable from a few second to one hour or more depending on the formulation. Several methods to determine the life of the foam include:

(i)   Visual inspection

(ii) Time for a given mass to penetrate the foam

(iii) Time for a given rod to fall which is inserted into the foam.

(iv) Rotational viscometers

VI. *Particle size determination:* Determination of particle size can be done by:

(i)   By Cascade impactor

(ii) By Light scatter decay

4. Biological Testing

This consists of determination of the therapeutic efficacy and toxicity.

Newer developments

1. There has been much interest in developing metered dose inhalers for a variety of conditions including Asthma, emphysema, diabetes, cancer, heart diseases, cystic fibrosis, etc.

2. A variable dose valve for administering insulin through nasal route is currently under development along with different, propellants, actuators.

26

Examination, Description and Sketching of Parts of an Aerosol Packaging System

Requirements: Container, valve assembly, opener etc.

Reference: Refer any book given in the list of books at the beginning of this manual.

Principle

Aerosol package consists of, usually a metal can or plastic bottle, designed to dispense its liquid contents as a mist or foam. The most common type of aerosol container consists of a shell, a valve, a "dip tube" that extends from the valve to the liquid product, and a liquefied-gas propellant under pressure. The liquid product is generally mixed with the propellant. When the valve is opened, this solution moves up the dip tube and out the valve. The propellant vaporizes as it is released into the atmosphere, dispersing the product in the form of fine particles.

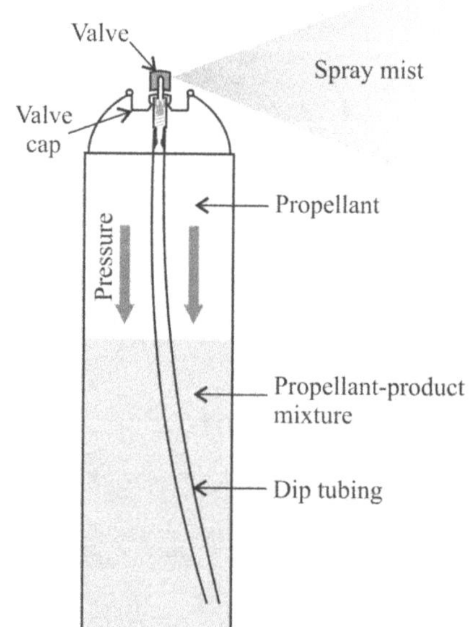

Fig. 26.1 Diagram of a typical aerosol container.

An aerosol dosage form consists of a number of components, which includes:

1. Containers
2. Valves assembly
3. Propellant
4. Product concentrate

1. Containers

They can be classified mainly in two categories. Detailed classification is given below.

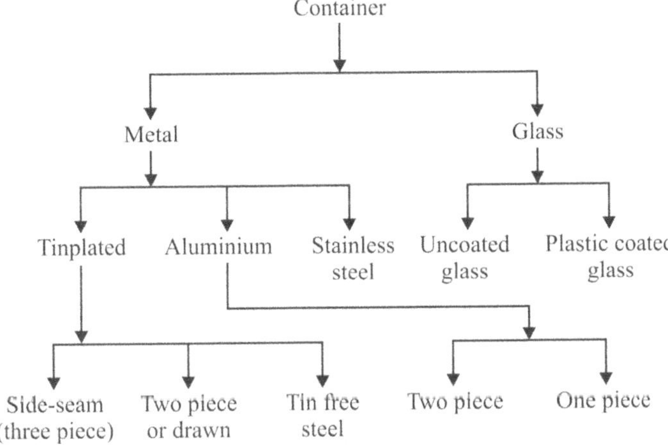

A. Metallic container:

(i) Tin plated Steel:

(a) Light weight and inexpensive steel.

(b) The addition of water and other corrosive ingredients or other substances, which will attack tin, requires a container having an additional coating.

(c) This coating is usually organic in nature and may consist of an oleoresin, phenolic, vinyl or epoxy coating.

(d) The liner (single or double coat) is added to the container prior to fabrication, (it is applied to the flat sheet of tin plate).

(e) Recent development in metal tin plate container is welded side seam –sudronic system and conoweld system

(ii) Aluminium: Used to manufacture extruded (seamless) aerosol container Greater resistance to corrosion.

(a) Lessened danger of incompatibility due to its seamless nature.

(b) Added resistance can be obtained by coating the inside of the container with organic materials such as epoxy, vinyl or phenolic resins.

(iii) Stainless Steel:

(a) These containers are limited to smaller sizes owing to production problems as well as cost.

(b) Extremely strong and resistant to most materials.

(c) No internal organic coating is required.

(iv) Glass: Available with or without coating.

(a) Incompatible.

(b) Non-corrosive in nature.

(c) Greater degree of freedom in design of the container.

e.g. Pharmaceutical and medicinal glass.

Two types of glass container are available

(a) Uncoated: Decreased cost and high clarity. The contents can be viewed at all times.

(b) Coated: Glass container is protected by plastic coating (plastic coated glass container) which prevents the glass from sheltering ring in the event of breakage.

2. Valves Assembly

There are two types of aerosol valves. They are:

(i) Continuous spray valves

(ii) Metered valves

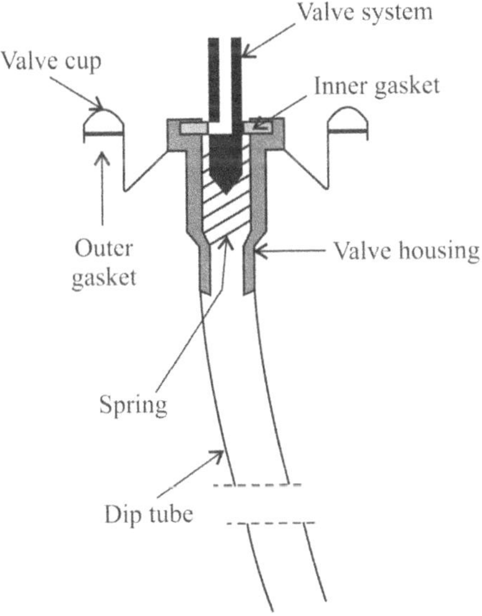

Fig. 26.2 Valve assembly.

Pharmaceutical valves should be:

(a) Easily opened and closed.

(b) Capable of delivering the content in the desired form.

(c) Deliver a given amount of medication.

(d) Constructed of material approved by Food and Drug Administration (FDA).

e.g.: spray foams and solid stream

Continuous spray valves: These valve assemblies consist of the following parts:

A. Actuators

- Activate the valve assembly and permits the easy opening and closing of the valve and is an integral part of almost every aerosol package.

- It is through the orifice in the actuator that the product is discharged.

- Design of inner chamber and size of the emission orifice of the actuator contribute to the physical form (mist, coarse spray, solid stream or foam)

- The particle size of emitted product can be controlled by combination, type, quantity of propellant used and actuator design and dimensions.
- It provides a rapid and convenient means for releasing the contents from pressured container.
- It provides the additional functional use in allowing the product to be dispersed in desired form i.e., fine moist wet spray, foam, or solid stream.

e.g., Metered dose inhalers.

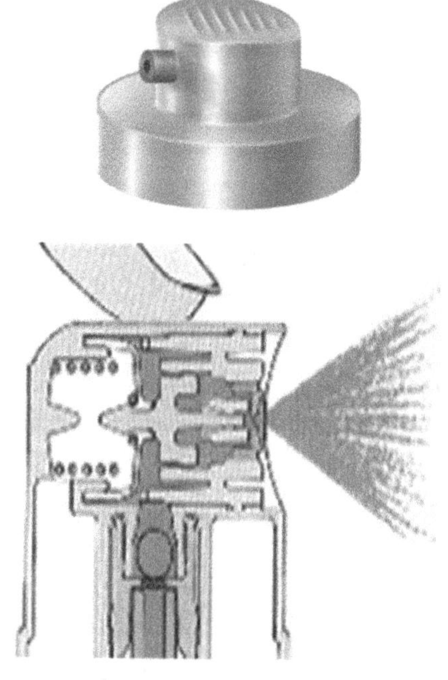

Fig. 26.3 Actuators.

Types: foam, spray, solid stream, special actuator for nose, throat etc.

B. Stem

(a) Supports the actuator.

(b) Delivers the formulation in the proper form to the chamber of the actuator.

(c) One or more orifices are set into the stem.

e.g. Nylon/metal (brass or stainless steel)

Fig. 26.4 Stem

C. Gasket

(a) Buna-N and Neoprene rubber are commonly used for gasket material.

(b) Compatible with most pharmaceutical product.

(c) Serves to prevent leakage of the formulation when the valve is in the closed position.

D. Spring

(a) Serves to hold gasket in place, when actuator is depressed and released. It returns the valve to its closed position.

e.g., Stainless steel can be used with most aerosols

E. Mounting Cup/Ferrule

(a) Used to attach the valve proper to container.

(b) Underside of the valve cup is exposed to the content of containers, single or double epoxy or vinyl coating can be added to increase resistance to corrosion.

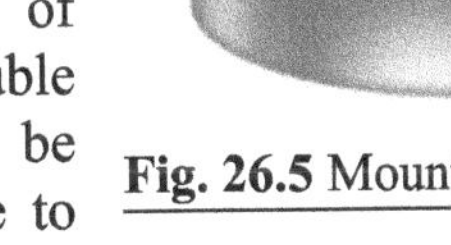

Fig. 26.5 Mounting cup.

e.g., Tinplate steel or aluminium

F. Housing/Valve Body

(a) Located directly below the mounting cup.

(b) Serves as the link between the dip tube stem and actuator.

(c) Made of nylon/delrin.

G. Dip Tube

- Extends from housing down into the product serves to bring the formulation from the container to the valve.

- Inside diameter is 0.120 to 0.125 inches and for highly viscous product the diameter is 0.195 inches.

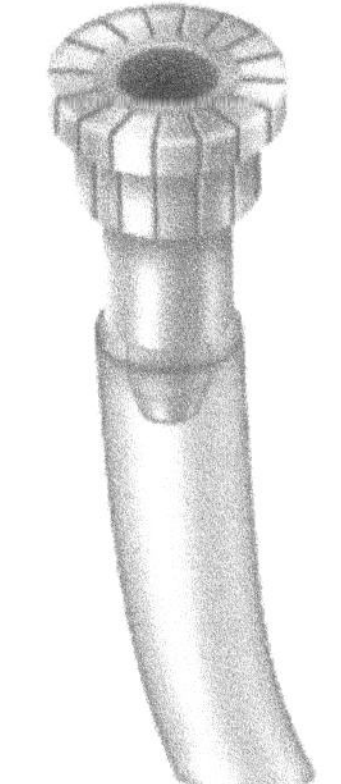

The selection of dip tube depends on

1. Viscosity of formulation.
2. Desired delivery rate.

Fig. 26.6 Dip tube and housing.

Functions: The tube serves several purposes.

(a) It conveys the liquid from the bottom of the container to the dispensing valve of the top.

(b) It prevents the propellant from escaping without dispensing the contents of the package.

H. Metering Valves

- Applicable to the dispensing of potent medication.
- Approx 50 to 150 mg ± 10% liquid material can be dispensed at time with the use of such valves.

Result: Different components of aerosol package were enumerated and studied.

3. Propellant

It is generally regarded as the heart of the aerosol package. In addition to supplying the necessary force to expect the product, it also act as solvent and diluent. It is responsible to develop proper pressure within the container to deliver the product.

Classification:

A. Liquefied Gases

Liquefied propellants are gases that exist as liquids under pressure

Ex: Fluorinated chlorinated hydrocarbons (halocarbons)

Hydrochlorofluocarbons, Hydrochlorocarbons, Hydorocarbons (Propane, butane and isobitane)

B. Compressed Gases

Ex: N_2, CO_2, N_2O

Selection of propellent is based on its boiling point, vapour pressure and density. The vapor pressure of a mixture of propellants can be calculated according to Daltons law "the total pressure in any system is equal to the sum of the individual or partial pressure of various components.

4. Product Concentrate

The product concentrate is the active ingredient or drug of the aerosol dosage form, which along with the required additives like, propellant, antioxidant, solvent, surfactants, suspending agents etc. is put in aerosol container . Depending on the nature of additives, the product concentrate may be of following types:

A. Solution Aerosols

Solution aerosols are two phase systems consisting of the product concentrate in a propellant or mixture of propellants or a mixture of propellant and solvent. Some solvents like Ethyl alcohol propylene glycol may also be added to the formulation to retard the evaporation of the propellant.

B. Suspension Aerosols

Suspension aerosols can prepare, when the product concentrate is insoluble in the propellant or mixture of propellant and solvent. Anti-asthmatic drugs, steroids and antibiotics are prepared in suspension aerosols.

C. Emulsion Aerosols

Emulsion aerosols consists of the active ingredient, surfactant/s, nonaqueous and/or aqueous vehicle/s. Depending on the components, the emitted product can be a stable foam (shaving cream type) or a quick breaking foam.

D. Foams

Foams can be produced when the product concentrate is dispersed in throughout the propellant and the propellant acts as the internal phase and in such cases o/w type of emulsion will form. While when the propellant is in the external phase, w/o emulsion will form and final product will expel in the form of sprays or wet streams .

Basic Principle to Release Product Concentrate from Container

Liquefied propellant or propellant mixture exists in equilibrium with the product concentrate in a sealed aerosol container. The liquefied propellant vapourises and occupies the upper portion of the aerosol container and exists in equilibrium with the propellant in the vapour phase in an aerosol container, so a constant pressure is maintained within the aerosol container. Hence, it is called as "a pressurised aerosol container". The pressure exerted by the propellant is called as "vapour pressure", measured in psig, is the characteristic of specific propellant. Upon the actuation of the valve, the pressure exerted by the propellant is distributed equally in all direction in the aerosol container, forcing the product concentrate up the dip tube and out of the aerosol container. As the vapour pressure of the propellant in air is lower than inside the aerosol container, propellant evaporates on reaching the air and product concentrates dries up in the form of dry particles.

27

Preparation and Evaluation of an Aerosol Dosage Form of Sulfanilamide

Requirements: Pestle-mortar, aerosol container, aerosol valve assembly, chemicals, propellant filling machine, valve crimping machine .

Reference: Refer any book given in the list of books at the beginning of this manual.

Formula

S. No.	Excipients	Quantity Given (gm)	Quantity Taken
1.	Silver Sulfanilamide	2	
2.	Benzocaine	2	
3.	PEG-400	2	
4.	Oleic Acid	2	
5.	PVP K30	2	
6.	Isopropyl alcohol	25	
7.	Propellant 11/12 (30:70)	59	

Principle

A successful aerosol formulation requires equipments, skills and knowledge as the manufacturing and the packaging operation are carried out simultaneously. This necessitates special quality control measures during the filling operations in order to ensure that both concentrate and propellant are brought together in the proper proportion. In general the manufacturing of aerosol product takes place in two stages.

Stage **I:** Manufacturing of the concentrate

Stage **II:** Addition of propellant.

On the laboratory scale, aerosol can be manufactured by any of the following methods.

Methods of Aerosol Filling

Cold filling method: In cold filling method, the product is chilled to – 40 °F and filled in chilled container followed by the addition of chilled propellant.

Pressure filling method: In this method the product pre-concentrate is filled in the container and valves are crimped in place, followed by the addition of propellant through valve under pressure.

Compressed gas filling: In this method, the product pre-concentrate is filled in the container and the valve is crimped. The air of the container is then removed by application of vacuum pump. The compressed gas is filled under pressure in the end.

In the present experiment pressure filling method was used to prepare a solution type aerosol using isopropyl alcohol and PEG-400 as solvent, propellant 11/12 as propellant, silver sulfanilamide (anti-bacterial) and benzocaine (local anaesthetic) as active ingredients. Use of oleic acid and PVP K30 is to sustain the action of the drugs at the site of application. Formulation then undergoes quality control tests and evaluated for various *in-vitro* and *in-vivo* parameters.

Procedure

- Dissolve polymer, oleic acid, benzocaine etc., in isopropyl alcohol.
- Mix sulfanilamide to above solution with continuous trituration.
- Continue triturating till a uniform suspension is obtained.
- Transfer the product to an aerosol bottle. Crimp the valve over the neck and fill the propellant to make its weight up to 50.0 g.
- Evaluate the product for following parameters.

Evaluation of Aerosol Dosgae Form

1. **Leak test:** Immerse each individual container in a bath of hot water maintained at 45-50°C for 3-5 minutes, so that contents reach the temperature of 45-50°C. Examine for any air bubble arising out of water. If no air bubbles arise, it indicates that valves and caps are properly crimped and there is no leakage.

2. **Delivery rate from container:** Immerse the container in a water bath at $21\pm1°C$ for half an hour (time required for the contents to reach that temperature). Remove the container from the water bath. Discharge for approximately 5 seconds to remove water and non-homogenous mixtures from the valve and dip tube. Wipe, dry and weigh the container. Hold the valve and open for 5 seconds and reweigh. Take the difference in weight and calculate delivery rate as loss in weight/second. Repeat it three times and calculate the average delivery rate as follows

Observations

- Weight of aerosol container preparation = **A gm**
- Weight of aerosol container after discharge for ' t' seconds = **B gm**
- Loss in weight /t seconds = A – B/t = **C gm/second**

    't' = 1,2,3-----time in minutes or seconds

3. **Film characteristics:** Clean the skin of the arm with water and soap and dry it with a towel. Spray the contents of each container on the skin of the arm and observe the film characteristics after 15 minutes and record the observation.

4. **Sensitivity test:** It is also known as open diagnostic patch test. Perform the test on the most sensitive part of the skin (inside bend of an elbow). Apply the aerosol formulation on about one square inch of the skin and leave it uncovered. The sites of patch were observed at the end of 24 hours and record the observations for hypersensitivity reaction, irritation or any other change on the skin.

5. **Flammability test:** Perform this test according to Australian flame projection test. Take a candle and burn it. Spray aerosol formulation 18 inches from the flame, and observe the extension of the flame and note down the readings.

Results:

The aerosol dosage form of silver sulfanilamide is prepared and evaluated for following parameters:

1. **Leak Test:** Passed/Failed.

2. **Delivery rate from each container:** _______ grams/seconds

3. **Film characteristics:** Uniform/Brittle/Thick/Thin ________.

4. **Sensitivity Test:** Passed / Failed.

5. **Flammability test:** Flame extension was found to be ________ cm.

Precautions

1. Crimping of valve should done carefully.
2. Flammability test should perform carefully.

PHARMA TRIVIA: SELF EVALUATION TEST

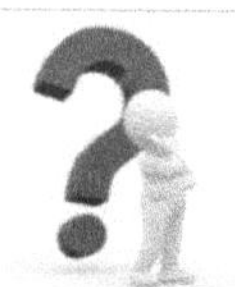

1. What are the components of aerosol package?

2. Describe briefly the materials used in manufacturing of aerosol containers.

3. Discuss about the propellants used in aerosols.

4. Mention the different types of valves used in pharmaceutical aerosol?

5. Write briefly about the actuators.

6. What are the types of systems used in pharmaceutical aerosol?

7. What are the Intra-nasal Aerosols?

8. Discuss briefly about the small-scale equipment used in the manufacturing of Pharmaceutical Aerosol.

9. Describe briefly about the industrial scale equipment for the manufacturing of Aerosols.

10. Write a brief note on the quality control testing procedure for pharmaceutical aerosols.

11. Discuss about the physicochemical testing used in evaluation of pharmaceutical aerosols

12. What are the different biological tests used to evaluate the pharmaceutical aerosols?

13. Define the terms – net contents, flame extension, spray pattern and foam stability.

14. Draw the well labelled diagram of an aerosol package and aerosol valve assembly.

15. Explain briefly the drug content tests for aerosols?

9

Modified Release Drug Delivery System

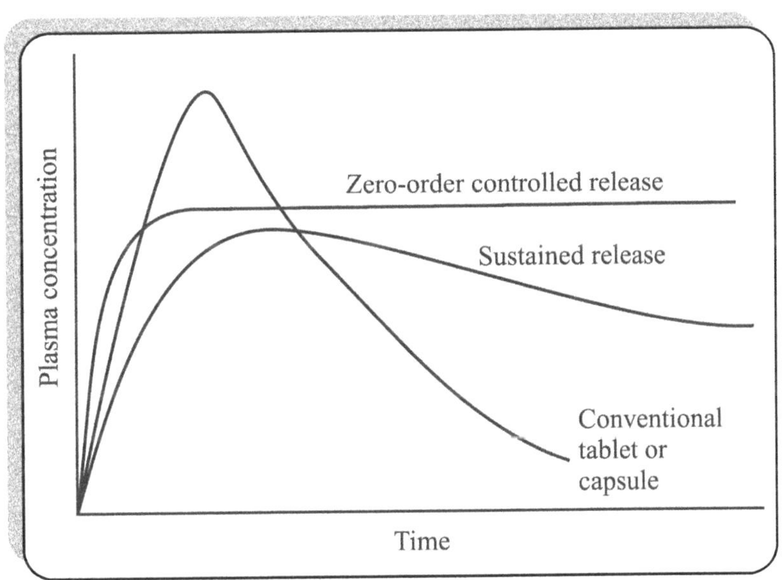

The term Ideal drug delivery system refered to a system which deliver the required amount of drug for particular period of time. Development of drug delivery system comprises of following steps

1. Preformulation study of drug
2. Formulation development
3. Medical device /technology to carry the formulation inside the body
4. Mechanism of release

Drug delivery systems are mainly divided into two types-**Immediate Release System and Modified Release System.** Immediate release system releases the drug immediately after administration. The other synonyms release like fast/conventional/Traditional release system can be used to define this system. While modified release dosage forms releases drug in modified manner or mostly in a sustained way. The other terms like slow/sustained/modern/extended drug delivery system can be used to define this system. The basic need of making oral modified release dosage forms is to release the drug at constant rate and at a desired site of action for extended period of time in order to achieve desired therapeutic benefits and patient compliance.

The MR dosage forms is divided into extended-release (ER) and delayed-release (DR) products. A DR dosage form releases a drug (or drugs) in a delayed   manner means after few hours of administration and often represented by lag time and graph will never starts from zero while an ER dosage form releases the drug over an extended period of time after administration, thus allowing a reduction in dosing frequency and dose related side effects compared to a drug given in conventional dosage form

Therapeutic Benefits of Modified Release Dosage Forms

- Reduction in frequency of dosage form administration
- Elimination of "surge and ebb" type of profile
- Reduction of total amount of drug needed to obtain   desired therapeutic response
- Reduction of incidence and degree of toxic or side effects
- Better patient compliance
- More efficient utilization of the drug in the body

- Reduction of irritation of gastrointestinal tract(GIT) caused by some orally administered drug

Limitations of Modified Release dosage forms

- Poor *in vitro-in vivo* correlation
- Possibility of dose dumping is high
- Retrieval of drug is difficult in case of poisoning
- Higher cost of formulation
- Stability Problems
- Increased variability among dosage units
- More rapid development of tolerance

Drug Candidate Criteria

All drugs are not suitable to design modified release dosage form. Only certain drugs with special characteristics are appropriate candidates for modified-release products. Following are some important properties that one should consider before selecting drug for designing of modified release dosage form

1. *Biological half life*: Drug having a very short biological half-life such as less than two hours is not a suitable candidate as it will require much larger dose achieve constant therapeutic blood levels throughout the day. In contrast to this, drug with long biological half life (>8hrs) is inherently sustained release and will remain in the body for extended period of time (5 times of the elimination half life ie approximately for 40 hrs) and therefore making a sustained release system of such drug will not be useful as the drug will already present in the body for a prolonged period of time. Hence drug having biological half-life between 2 to 8 hours or more appropriately 3to 4 hours considered to be an ideal candidate for modified release formulation.

2. *Therapeutic range*: Therapeutic range should be moderate. The drug should possess a good margin of safety so if dose dumping occurs the drug concentration level cannot go beyond toxic levels that could be harmful to the patient. Moreover formulator can also free to try wide range of dose for optimization.

3. *GI absorption*: The drugs which show uniform absorption throughout the GI tract (from the stomach to the colon) are good candidates. It should not show any absorption window or pH

dependant absorption otherwise it will be difficult to maintain sustained drugs levels for desired period as no drug absorption will occur at particular parts in the GI tract.

4. *Aqueous solubility*: Highly soluble and poorly soluble drugs are not ideal candidates. If solubility of drug is very poor, absorption of such drugs will be dissolution limited and hence designing of sustained release formulation of such drug will further sustained the blood level resulting in more delayed therapeutic response which ultimately lead to patient noncompliance. On the other hand if the solubility is very high then it will be very difficult to decrease its dissolution rate. Therefore drug requires moderate solubility.

5. *Stability*: Selected drug should be stable against wide pH range, GI enzyme and microbial flora of GI tract

6. *Dose*: Dose of drug should be small. Potent drugs with moderate therapeutic window are considered to be good candidates for modified release dosage forms. The main purpose of Modified release dosage form is to reduce the dose frequency to the level where single daily dose in form one tablet or capsule is sufficient to maintain constant drug level throughout the day. If dose is very high then the size of tablet or capsule may be too large for the patient to swallow and if by mistake patient chews the tablet/capsule and dose dumping may occurs and drug concentration will go beyond the toxic level that could be hrmful to the patient. On the other hand if dose is small abovementioned problems may not occure.

7. *Absorption and elimination*: Rate of absorption and elimination of drug should be moderate. If the absorption rate is too slow, then the onset of therapeutic action will be very slow which ultimately retard release rate.

8. *Disease state*: Modified release dosage forms are useful in the treatment of chronic diseases rather than acute conditions. Acute conditions always require immediate release of drug while in chronic conditions requires slow and constant blood level for extended period of time.

Types of Oral Modified Release Dosage Forms

  I. Extended release system

      A. Diffusion controlled system

          (i) Membrane/Reservoir type (Coated/encapsulated type)

         (ii) Matrix type (mixture type)

    B. Dissolution controlled system
- (i) Reservoir type.
- (ii) Matrix type

    C. Ion exchange resin

    D. Osmotic pump

    E. pH independent formulations

    F. Slow dissolving salts and complexes

    G. Gastro- retentive Drug delivery System
- (i)   Altered density
- (ii) Size based system
- (iii) Mucoadhesive system

    H. Pulsatile Release system

    I. Bimodal/Biphasic release system

II. Delayed Release system

    A. Enteric coated system

    B. Colonic Release system

Rate-Controlling Materials (Film Formers)

Polymer is an integral part of modified release dosage form and wide varieties of polymers are available to optimize the rate of drug delivery. Type of polymer, their combination and concentration are key factors to provide desired modulation in drug release. For hydrophilic matrix systems natural polymers such as xantham gum and alginate, semisynthetic polymers like hydroxypropyl methylcellulose (HPMC), sodium CMC, Hydroxypropyl cellulose, synthetic polymer such as Poly (vinyl chloride), poly (vinyl pyrrolidone) and poly(methacrylic acid) of varying degree of cross-linking, are available. Some of these polymers such as alginate and poly(methacrylic acid) are polyelectrolytes in nature and used in preparation of varies novel drug delivery systems with unique release-modifying properties.

For hydrophobic matrix system insoluble polymers such as Eudragit RL, RS, polyvinylacetate ethyl cellulose, cellulose acetate, and other cellulose esters can be used. Fatty acids and their various glycerol esters and wax-like materials have also been used previously.

Polymers like cellulose acetate, cellulose derivatives such as ethyl cellulose and cellulose butyrate provide semi-permeable membrane coating and are most commonly used in osmotic pump preparation.

Enteric polymers which dissolve at higher pHs are used in delayed release preparations. Enteric coating is generally used for drugs showing instability in acidic environment or when action is required in intestine or drug shows absorption window in intestine. The enteric coating may be

- *pH dependent*: breaking down in the less acidic environment of the intestine,

- *Time dependent*: eroding by moisture over time during gastrointestinal transit,

- *Enzyme dependent*: degrading slowly as a result of the hydrolysis-catalyzing action of intestinal enzymes.

Based on drug properties and design objectives different polymers, (single or in combination) at particular concentrations may be used to make the drug release in intestine for extended period. For example, Eudragit L 55 is soluble at pH > 5.5; Eudragit L 100, is soluble at pH > 6. Eudragit S (100) is soluble at pH > 7. Polymers commonly used for enteric coating are shellac, Zein and cellulose Phthalate polymers (cellulose acetate phthalate, methyl cellulose phthalate), Cellulose acetate butyrate etc. These polymers may be used alone or in combination to achieve a predetermined release delay.

USP Requirements and FDA Guidance for Modified-Release Dosage Forms

The following tests are important for quality control of modified release dosage forms

1. **Drug release**

    The drug release for extended-release and delayed-release products is based on drug dissolution from the dosage unit against elapsed test time.

Time (hr)	Amount dissolved
1.0	between 15% and 40%
2.0	between 25% and 60%
4.0	between 35% and 75%
8.0	not less than 70%

2. Uniformity of dosage units

It is determined by two methods

1. Weight variation test
2. Content uniformity test.

3. *In vitro/in vivo* correlations (IVIVCs)

IVIVCs is a decisive step in the development of oral extended-release products and it is monitored throughout the periods of product development, clinical evaluation, submission of an application for FDA-approval for marketing, and during postapproval for any formulation or manufacturing changes which are proposed.

28

To Prepare and Evaluate Control Release Tablet of Paracetamol

Requirements: Pestle mortar, Sieves (# 8, 20, 44), Filter paper sheets, Hardness tester, Friabilator.

Reference: Refer any book given in the list of books at the beginning of this manual.

Formula:

For 300 mg tablet.

S. No.	Ingredients	Quantity per tablet			
		F1[*]	F2[*]	F3[*]	F4[*]
1.	Paracetamol	100 mg	100 mg	100 mg	100 mg
2.	HPMC	50 mg	50 mg	100 mg	100 mg
3.	PVP K 30	40 mg	80 mg	40 mg	80 mg
4.	Talc	2.5 mg	2.5 mg	2.5 mg	2.5 mg
5.	Magnesium stearate	1.5mg	1.5mg	1.5 mg	1.5 mg
6.	MCC	106 mg	66 mg	56 mg	16 mg

[*]Calculate the quantities for 25 tablets.

Principle

Use of conventional drug delivery systems suffers with number of limitations such as frequent dosing, severe side effects and no precise control over the maintenance of plasma levels of drug resulting into the poor patient compliance. Such limitations leading to the development of novel drug delivery systems with controlled and desired release characteristics. In conventional drug delivery system the rate of release of medicament from the dosage form is fast and absorption is the rate (Ka) limiting factor. While in the controlled drug delivery systems the release of the medicament from the dosage form is very slow and hence release rate constant (Kr) is a rate limiting factor. Various types of control release systems include:

- **Delayed release** indicates that the drug is not being released immediately following administration but after a certain time interval (lag time) e.g., entericcoated tablets, pulsatile-release capsules.

- **Repeat action** indicates that an individual dose is released fairly soon after administration, and second or third doses are subsequently released at intermittent intervals.

- **Prolonged release** indicates that the drug is provided for absorption over a longer period of time than from a conventional dosage form. However, there is an implication that onset is delayed because of an overall slower release rate from the dosage form.

- **Sustained release** indicates an initial release of drug sufficient to provide a therapeutic dose soon after administration (loading dose), and then a gradual release over an extended period (maintenance dose).

There are various types of control release dosage forms available such as transdermal, implantables, transmucosal, oral controlled and parenteral controlled. Various types of the polymers are used for their preparations such as: natural (chitosan, alginates etc.), semi-synthetic (ethyl cellulose, HPMC etc.) and synthetic polymers (PVP, PLA, PLGA etc.).

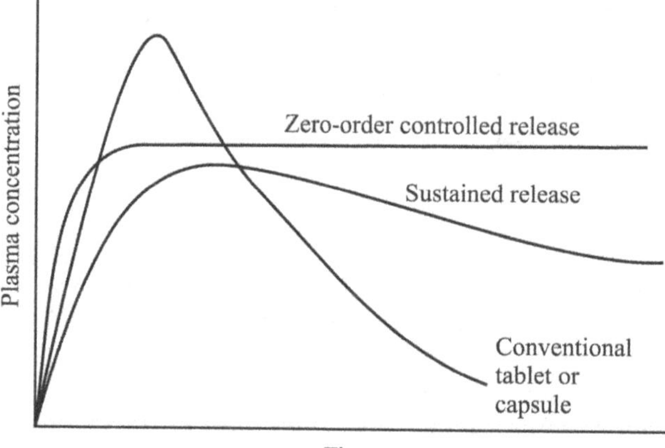

In the present experiment controlled release tablet of paracetamol is prepared by the aqueous wet granulation method. HPMC, CMC and PVP K 30 are used as release retardant polymer (Sustain release polymers). Talc and magnesium stearate are used as glidants.

Procedure

Calculate the quantity of each excipient for 25 tablets. Weigh and mix all excipients except talc and magnesium stearate. Make a dough with the help of water or alcohol. Rest of the procedure is same as experiment no 12

Evaluation: As per experiment no 9, except the disintegration test.

Storage: Store in a well closed containers in a cool dry place.

Category: Analgcsic, antipyrctic.

Results: As per experiment no. 9.

Note: Disintegration test is not performed on controlled release tablets.

To Prepare and Evaluate Solid Dispersion of Sulphanilamide

Requirements: Sulphanilamide, PEG 6000, methanol, beakers, glass rods, dissolution apparatus, funnel, stand, measuring cylinders, pipette etc.

Reference: Refer any book given in the list of books at the beginning of this manual.

Formula

S. No.	Formulation Code	Drug	Polymer (PEG 6000)
1.	F1	1 gm	0.5 gm
2.	F2	1 gm	1 gm
3.	F3	1 gm	1.5 gm
4.	F4	1 gm	2 gm

Principle

The term solid dispersion refers to a group of solid products consisting of at least two different components, generally a hydrophilic matrix and a hydrophobic drug. The matrix can be either crystalline or amorphous. The drug can be dispersed molecularly, in amorphous particles (clusters) or in crystalline particles.

Advantages of solid dispersion

1. Particles with reduced size
2. Particles with improved wettability
3. Particles with higher porosity
4. Drugs in amorphous state

Preparation of solid dispersions

- *Fusion method*: The melting or fusion method is the preparation of physical mixture of a drug and a water-soluble carrier and heating it directly until it melts. The melted mixture is then solidified rapidly in an ice-bath under vigorous stirring. The final solid mass is crushed, pulverized and sieved.

- *Solvent method*: In this method, the physical mixture of the drug and carrier is dissolved in a common solvent, which is evaporated until a clear, solvent free film is left. The film is further dried to constant weight.

- *Melting solvent method* (*melt evaporation*): It involves preparation of solid dispersions by dissolving the drug in a suitable liquid solvent and then incorporating the solution directly into the melt of polyethylene glycol, which is then evaporated until a clear, solvent free film is left. The film is further dried to constant weight.

- *Melt extrusion method*: The drug/carrier mix is typically processed with a twin screw extruder. The drug/carrier mix is simultaneously melted, homogenized and then extruded and shaped as tablets, granules, pellets, sheets, sticks or powder. The intermediates can then be further processed into conventional tablets.

- *Lyophilization Technique*: Lyophilization involves transfer of heat and mass to and from the product under preparation. This technique was proposed as an alternative technique to solvent evaporation.

- *Super Critical Fluid (Scf) Technology*: The supercritical fluid antisolvent techniques, carbon dioxide are used as an antisolvent for the solute but as a solvent with respect to the organic solvent.

Procedure

- Solid dispersion of sulphanilamide and PEG is prepared by melt evaporation method.

- Take the required amount of sulphanilamide and dissolve in methanol.

- Melt the PEG 6000 at 50-60 °C and then add it to the drug solution and mix thoroughly.

- Keep the obtained mixture at 50-60 °C for 72 h and then cool the solution at room temperature to form a solid.

- The prepared solid dispersion is then passed through sieve no. 40.
- Prepare the solid dispersion of the different formula in the similar manner.

Evaluation of the Solid Dispersion

Flow Properties

As per experiment no. 7.

Dissolution studies

Perform the dissolution studies using dissolution apparatus I (IP) as per the experiment no. 6 compare the dissolution profile of different formulations with the marketed preparation containing equivalent amount of sulphanilamide.

Results: Solid dispersion of sulphanilamide was prepared and angle of repose, bulk density were found to be _________ and _________ respectively.

Dissolution studies showed the dissolution is slower/faster from the solid dispersion than the marketed preparation.

PHARMA TRIVIA: SELF EVALUATION TEST

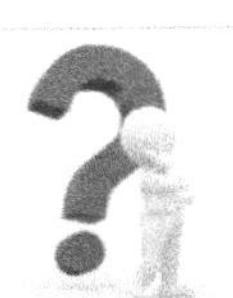

1. Define the following terms:
   (a) Controlled/ Temporal drug delivery system
   (b) Sustained drug delivery system
   (c) Extended release systems
   (d) Delayed release systems
   (e) Spatial / site specific/ targeted drug delivery system

2. Give the examples of each:
   (a) Water insoluble polymers
   (b) Hydrophilic polymers
   (c) Enteric coated polymers
   (d) Biodegradable polymers

3. What are the advantages and disadvantages of controlled drug delivery systems?

4. What are ocuserts?

5. What do you understand by the term transdermal drug delivery system?

6. Classify parenteral controlled drug delivery systems.

7. List various oral controlled release systems.

8. Define biodegradable polymers with suitable examples.

9. Give examples of hydrophilic polymers.

10. Give examples of pH sensitive polymers.

11. Define AUC & absolute bioavailability.

12. What are the applications of solid dispersions?

13. Give two examples of solubility enhancing agents.

14. What are the various methods of preparing solid dispersions?

15. Name any two polymers used in solid dispersions?

10

Packaging System

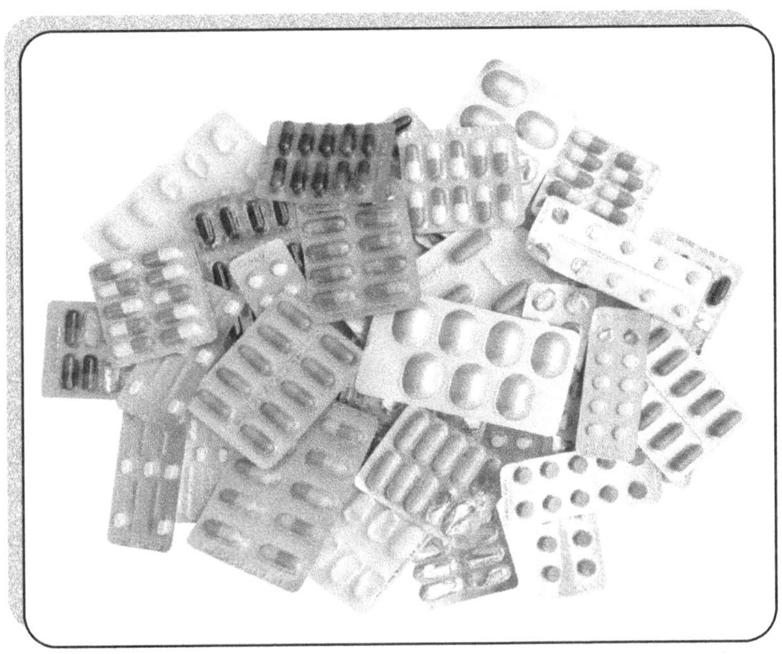

INTRODUCTION

A product is not correctly formulated unless it is properly packaged, and in some cases the major part of the formulation process may be concerned with selecting the right package for the product. The stability of the pharmaceutical may be totally dependent on proper functioning of the package, for e.g., there must be rigorous exclusion of light and oxygen from oily vitamin preparation if loss of potency due to oxidation is to be avoided.

Packaging is the means of providing protection, presentation, identification, information, containment and convenience/compliance for the product during storage, transport, display and use. Ideally, no interaction should occurr between product and package. In modern era of technology the package and dosage have commonly become so intertwined that the drug product itself must be defined in terms of both package and formulation. Some specific examples are - transdermal patch, metered dose inhalers prefilled syringes and nasal sprays all contain formulations whose quantity and successful delivery are strongly dependent upon the proper function of the package system. In the above context, pharmaceutical packaging may be defined as - the combination of components necessary to contain, preserve, protect and deliver drug product safely and effectively.

The pack may be usually present in up to three layers:

1. **Primary pack** or immediate packaging are those that are in direct contract with the product being packed; the container should not interact physically or chemically with the contents

2. **Secondary pack,** for information and additional protection and they are not in direct contact with the product

3. **Tertiary pack,** for storage and distribution

   Secondary and tertiary packs together are sometimes referred as Ancillary pack.

The design of a package depends upon many criteria, such as

- The type of product
- Route of administration of the product
- Available material and their compatibility with the product
- Available equipment to achieve the final pack

- Method of assembling the pack
- How the proof of consistency of production is achieved.

Following are some special types of primary packaging

(a) Child resistance packaging

(b) Tamper resistance packaging

(c) Compliance packaging

PACKAGING MATERIALS

With very few exceptions containers and closures are mainly fabricated from metals or rubber or plastic.

1. Plastic

Plastic is a light moldable material which is usually very resistant to breakage. Plastic packaging is used for bottles, jars, ampoules, closures, plugs, films, sheets, labels; shrink sleeves wads, cartons and tubing. Owing to the versatile properties, plastic films and laminates are being extremely used for packaging of wide variety of commodity. The plastics used in the containers consist of one or more polymers together with certain additives (eg., plasticizers, resins, stabilizers, lubricants, antistatic agents, mold release agents) if necessary. The nature of the additives is often dependent on the polymer composition and the method of manufacture of the plastic material. Opacifiers can also be added for protection of content from light.

Advantages

- Low cost
- light weight
- Ease of fabrication
- Reasonably high quality
- Freedom of design to which they lend themselves
- Extremely resistant to breakage and thus offer safety to consumer along with reduction of breakage losses at all levels of distribution and use.

Disadvantages

Drug plastic interaction may involve:

- Permeation

- Leaching
- Sorption
- Chemical reaction
- Alteration of the physical characteristics of the polymer of the product

The quality of plastic is governed by following parameters

- Chemical structure
- Molecular weight
- Crystallinity and orientation
- Cross linking
- Addition of other agents

2. Glass

Glass packaging includes bottles, vials, ampules, jars, vitrellae, cartridges and prefilled syringes. Glass is one of the earliest known packaging materials and even today glass containers are widely used in packaging. The attributes of glass relevant to consumer packaging are its chemical inertness, impermeability, transparency, strength, color, shape etc. It can be manufactured in any shape depending on the type of the product to be packed. Furthermore, by varying the chemical composition of glass, it is possible to adjust the chemical behavior and radiation protective properties of glass. Glass does not deteriorate with age and with proper closure system, it provides an excellent barrier against practically every element except light. The glass usable for pharmaceutical (including parenteral) packing has been classified by the USP/NF according to types based on the capability to resist hydrolytic attack.

Table 10.1 USP/NF Glass Classifications

Types	General description	Applications
I	Highly resistant borosilicate glass	• Water for injection • Unbuffered products • Products that are alkaline or will become alkaline prior to their expiration date
II	Treated soda-lime glass	• Products that remain below pH for their shelf life. • Large volume parenterals

Table 10.1 *Contd...*

Types	General description	Applications
III	Soda-lime glass	• Dry powders that are subsequently dissolved to make a buffered solution • Liquid formulations that are insensitive to alkali
IV	General purpose Soda-lime glass	• General purpose

Limitations of glass as packaging material

- Leaching and corrosion of glass surfaces in contact with water or aqueous solutions.
- The mechanical handling of the glassware, at both the glass manufacturer and the bottler, can damage the surface externally and internally.
- Formation of insoluble precipitates with time.
- Ability to adsorb active drug on the surface and thereby reduced potency.

3. Metal

Metal packaging includes rigid cylindrical tins, collapsible tubes, cans for aerosols, valves, closures and foils, mostly made of aluminum, tinplated steel, stainless steel, tin-free steel.

Advantages

- Metal is strong, opaque, and impermeable to moisture, odors, light, gases, liquids and biological contaminants.
- They can be easily coated to prevent the direct contact with the contents.
- It is also resistant to high and low temperature.

Limitations

- Metal is highly reactive and susceptible to corrosion in long term in the presence of oxygen, moisture, acids and alkalis. The corrosion can be prevented by coating or lacquering. Coating, however, presents additional problems, since coating material must be inert for preparation and it should completely cover the underlying material. In addition, the coating must be evaluated for resistance to cracking and solvents.
- Cost of some metals especially tin is relatively expensive.

4. Paper and Board

Paper and board packaging is used mainly for secondary and tertiary packaging. For examples - Labels, leaflets, cartons and cases. Various dressings, pouches and medical devices have paper as a contact material. Other packages using paper based materials are

- Wrapping materials
- Fiber drums
- Lined carton system
- Labels
- Sealing tapes
- Laminates
- Multiwall paper bags and sacs

Composition

Paper and board are composed of cellulose. The cellulose is obtained by the mechanical or semi-chemical treatment of vegetable fibers (pulp) derived from various sources like wood, hemp, and cotton etc. Waste and regenerated paper can also be used in some cases.

Advantages

- Non-toxic and environment friendly
- Low cost
- Reasonable strength and rigidity
- Printability
- Obtained from natural source

Limitations

- High permeability so coating/lamination may be required.
- Paper can be heat sealed only when coated
- Opacity
- Can be torn easily in the direction of grains
- Expands or contract with the absorption/release of moisture

30

To Evaluate the Given Packaging System

Requirements: Vernier caliper, packaging system (strip package), small glass beaker, vacuum assembly, cellophane tape.

Sample: Disprin Tablet strip packaging system

Reference: Refer any book given in the list of books at the beginning of this manual.

Principle

Packaging can be defined as an economical means of providing presentation, protection, identification/information, containment, convenience and compliance for a product during storage, carriage, display and use until such time as the product is used or administered.

Importance of packaging

- Protect against all adverse external influences that can alter the properties of the product.
- Protect against biological contamination.
- Protect against physical damage.
- Carry the correct information and identification of the product.
- Tamper evident / Child resistance / Anti counterfeiting.

Strip packs: It represents an alternative form of packaging for unit dose medication. It is formed by feeding two weds of a heat-sealable flexible film through either a heat crimping roller or a heat reciprocating platen. The product is dropped into the pocket prior to forming final set of seals. The product is sealed between the two sheets of film and usually has a seal around each tablet, with perforations usually separating adjacent packets. The pocket area is critical to diameter, shape and thickness. The pocket area is extended when the product is inserted. Strip designs are basically either square or in rectangular form. Strip packages are produced at lower speed and occupy greater volume than blister pack. The process is same as pouch packaging but on a smaller scale.

Different packaging materials are used for strip packaging. The selection of material depends on both product and equipment requirements. For high-barrier applications, a paper/polyethylene/foil/polyethylene lamination is commonly used. When product visibility is required heat sealable cellophane or heat sealable polyester can be used.

Procedure

The given packaging system is evaluated for the following parameters:

1. **Thickness Test:** Measure the thickness of the foil at different places of the strip using vernier caliper.

2. **Extractive Matter Test:**
   - Weigh accurately about 5 g of cut aluminum foil and put in a weighed beaker
   - Add 25 ml of acetone in it and stir the pieces of foil for 15-20 minutes.
   - Remove the foil pieces and wash them with 10 ml of acetone and add the washings to the original extract.
   - Evaporate to dryness and weigh the beaker again. Calculate the % age of extractable matter as follows-

   Weight of empty beaker = A gm

   Weight of beaker + Dried extractive material = B gms

   Weight of foil = S gm

   % Weight of extractive material

   $$= \frac{B - A\left(\text{weight of extract}\right) \times 100}{S\left(\text{weight of foil}\right)}$$

3. **Leak Test:**
   - Fold the intact strip containing tablets/capsules and put it into flask of vacuum assembly.

- Stopper the flask, connect the side opening to a filter pump and apply suction for 10 minutes.
- Retrieve the packaging material, open the pack and observe for the presence of moisture inside each packet.
- Moistening of the tablet or capsules inside, shows poor sealing or presence of pinholes and failure of test.

4. Quality of Printing:

- Affix a cellophane tape on the printed portion of the foil and peel it off to assess the quality of printing.
- If the print gets peeled off with the cellophane tape, it indicates poor quality of printing.

Results:

1. **Thickness** _______ mm.
2. **% Extractive material** _______ %.
3. **Leak Test:** passed /failed.
4. **Quality of printing:** satisfactory/ poor.

31

To Evaluate the Plastic Vials for their Moisture Transmission Property

Requirements: Desiccator, 15 plastic containers of uniform size,

Desiccant: Place a quantity of 4 mesh anhydrous calcium chloride in a shallow container, taking care to exclude any fine powder, then dry at 110 °C for 1 hour and cool in a dessicator.

Procedure

- Wcigh 12 containers of uniform size and type.
- Clean the sealing surfaces with lint free cloth and close and open each container 30 times.
- Apply the closure firmly and uniformly each time the container is closed.
- Add desiccant to 10 of the designated test containers up to two third of the volume.
- Close each container immediately after adding desiccant.
- To each of the remaining two containers, designated as controls add sufficient number of glass beads to attain a weight approximately equal to that of each of the test containers and close them firmly.
- Keep all the containers in a tight desiccators containing saturated solution of sodium chloride (35 g in 100 ml of water).
- After 14 days, record the weight of the individual containers in the same manner.

- Completely fill 5 empty containers under test with water to the level indicated by the closure surface when in place.
- Transfer the contents of each to a graduated cylinder, and determine the average container volume in ml.
- Calculate the rate of moisture permeability, in mg per day per liter by the formula:

$$\text{Rate of permeability of moisture} = 1000\left[\left(T_f - T_i\right) - \frac{\left(C_f - C_i\right)}{14V}\right]$$

Where

V = Volume in ml of the container

$(T_f - T_i)$ - Difference in mg between the final and initial weights of each test container.

$(C_f - C_i)$ - Average of the difference in mg between the final and initial weights of the 2 control containers.

- The containers so tested are tight containers if not more than one of the 10-test container exceeds 100 mg per day per litre in moisture permeability and none exceeds 200 mg per day litre.
- The containers are wheel closed containers is not more than one of the 10 test containers exceeds 2000 mg per day per litre in moisture permeability and none exceeds 3000 mg per day per litre.

Results: Rate of permeability of moisture is ------, therefore the test is passed/failed.

PHARMA TRIVIA: SELF EVALUATION TEST

1. Define an ideal packaging system.
2. Mention the various characteristics of an ideal packaging system.
3. Give the composition of glass I.
4. What is the significance of using Boron oxide, lead & aluminium oxide in the manufacturing of glass?
5. Enlist the various types of glasses as per USP.
6. What are the tests done for evaluating the chemical resistance of glass.
7. What do you mean by blooming/weathering?
8. Enlist various drug-plastic interactions.
9. Name the different types of closures.
10. Enlist the types of ingredients commonly found in a rubber closure.
11. Differentiate between thermosetting and thermoplastic materials.
12. Define tamper-resistant packaging.
13. Give examples of tamper resistant packaging systems.
14. Give the formulae for % extractive material.
15. Briefly explain the leak test for a strip packaging system.

www.ingramcontent.com/pod-product-compliance
Lightning Source LLC
LaVergne TN
LVHW081721210726
843527LV00005B/272